W9-BSA-815

THE PREPPER'S
GUIDE TO
SURVIVING
PANDEMICS,
BIOTERRORISM,
AND INFECTIOUS
DISEASE

THE PREPPER'S GUIDE TO SURVIVING PANDEMICS, BIOTERRORISM, AND INFECTIOUS DISEASE

WILLIAM W. FORGEY,
MD, FAWM, CCHP-P, CTH®

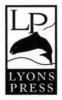

LYONS PRESS

Guilford, Connecticut

An imprint of Globe Pequot, the trade division of
The Rowman & Littlefield Publishing Group, Inc.
4501 Forbes Blvd., Ste. 200
Lanham, MD 20706
LyonsPress.com

Distributed by NATIONAL BOOK NETWORK

Illustrations by David R. Scott unless otherwise noted

British Library Cataloguing in Publication Information available

Library of Congress Cataloging-in-Publication Data available

Names: Forgey, William W., 1942– author.
Title: The prepper's guide to surviving pandemics, bioterrorism, and
  infectious disease / by William W. Forgey, MD, FAWM, CCHP-P, CTH.
Description: Guilford, Connecticut : Lyons Press, [2022] | Includes
  bibliographical references and index. | Summary: "Covers the pandemic
  caused by SARS-CoV-2 and also delves into the massive controversy
  concerning herd immunity, which vaccines are the most likely to work,
  the issue of second wave or resurgence caused by school reopenings and
  other activities, changes in public policy, and numerous other topics"—
  Provided by publisher.
Identifiers: LCCN 2021019059 (print) | LCCN 2021019060 (ebook) | ISBN
  9781493060511 (paperback) | ISBN 9781493060528 (epub)
Subjects: LCSH: Epidemics. | Bioterrorism. | Survival.
Classification: LCC RA648.5 .F67 2022 (print) | LCC RA648.5 (ebook) | DDC
  614.4—dc23
LC record available at https://lccn.loc.gov/2021019059
LC ebook record available at https://lccn.loc.gov/2021019060

♾™ The paper used in this publication meets the minimum requirements of American National Standard for Information Sciences—Permanence of Paper for Printed Library Materials, ANSI/NISO Z39.48-1992.

The health information expressed in this book is based solely on the personal experience of the author and is not intended as a medical manual. The information should not be used for diagnosis or treatment, or as a substitute for professional medical care.

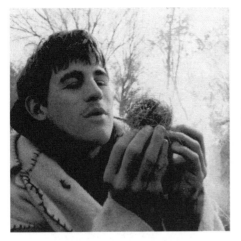

David R. Scott, circa 1992, while on his Arctic adventure.
IMAGE COURTESY DAVID R. SCOTT

This book is dedicated to my good friend and the illustrator of this book, David Ryan Scott. In 1992, at the age of 19, Dave and a friend of his, Scott Power, went into the subarctic wilderness of northern Canada on a trip that I sponsored. They built a cabin and spent a year—two winters and one summer. Their adventure has recently been republished by David as a Kindle book called *Paradise Creek*, which was originally a Globe Pequot publication now out of print. Since then, the two of them and I have traveled on numerous trips into wilderness areas all over the world. They have both been of great help in establishing my medical clinic in Haiti.

I particularly appreciate the help David has provided me on this and several of my books with his illustrations and advice.

CONTENTS

CHAPTER 1

THE COVID-19 SURVIVAL GUIDE

To make decisions—and more importantly, so you can understand comments and decisions provided you by governmental authorities—this book explains the basics about SARS-CoV-2 and Covid-19, the disease it causes, provides links to daily updated data, and describes past pandemics whose management we forget at our peril. This includes what these terrible natural disasters could become if they were turned into either purposeful or accidental bioterrorist weapons.

Early in this pandemic there was a significant setback when the disease became a political issue. This is not unusual with severe pandemics. They always result in tremendous political upheaval, lockdowns, resistance to lockdowns, even the collapse of societies and empires. In London during the Black Death, quarantine was strictly enforced by watchmen posted in front of any house with an infected individual inside. People were so desperate to escape from their homes they would carve through the walls, only to be beaten back by the ever-careful watchmen. And if the watchmen were not careful, they could fall prey to the noose. Confined home-dwellers were known to wait until the watchman nodded off asleep in front of their house, then lower a noose from the second floor around his neck, hanging him and thus making their break from confinement. There are reports of friends or family sneaking poison into the watchman's food or drink so the confined could escape. So the occasional scuffles between people wearing or not wearing masks seems tame in comparison to the historical upheaval that disease outbreaks have caused within a society. There's much more on this in the section on pandemics.

How do I know if I have Covid-19 or some other condition?
Covid-19 affects different people in different ways. Perhaps 40 percent will never develop symptoms but unfortunately can pass the disease to others. Most infected people will develop mild to moderate illness and recover without hospitalization.

What is the difference between isolation and quarantine?
Isolation is placing an ill person into a period of confinement, while quarantine is placing an exposed person into confinement. Oddly enough, the quarantine of an exposed person can last longer than the

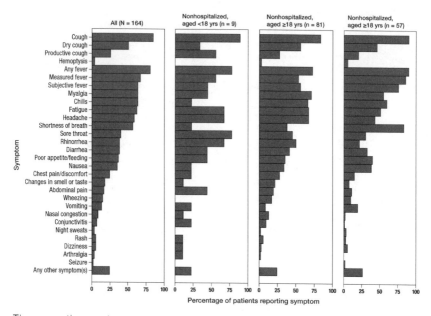

These are the most common symptoms at onset by severity of disease in those who are unlucky enough to progress to worse disease.

isolation of an ill person. Once ill, a person can get over a disease and no longer be contagious, while an exposed person may have a much longer period of time that they are incubating the illness and being contagious.

What is a quarantine period and how long should it last?

The ideal quarantine period should match the full incubation period so that nobody exposed to the disease, even those who are asymptomatic, can pass the disease on to others. Obviously, some people incubate the disease longer than others. It has been shown that some persons exposed to a Covid-19 patient did not develop the illness for 28 days, but this is an outlier. Initially, the median incubation period was estimated to be 5.1 days (the period when half of those infected was 4.5 to 5.8 days), and that 97.5 percent of those who developed symptoms did so within 11.5 days (95 percent confidence interval was 8.2 to 15.6 days) of exposure. These estimates imply that, under conservative assumptions, 101 out of every 10,000 cases (99th percentile) will develop symptoms after 14 days of active monitoring or quarantine.[1] So initially the quarantine period of persons exposed to SARS-CoV-2 was 14 days.

The term "quarantine," or in Italian, *quaranta giorni*, comes from the late medieval period when the plague resulted in the first official isolation of incoming ships, cargo, and people for 40 days. Thankfully, quarantine periods for Covid-19 have been much less.

One year into the pandemic (in February 2021), the US Centers for Disease Control and Prevention (CDC) released the following quarantine instructions:

> For most adults with COVID-19 illness, isolation and precautions can be discontinued 10 days after symptom onset and after resolution of fever for at least 24 hours, without the use of fever-reducing medications, and with improvement of other symptoms.
>
> Some adults with severe illness may produce replication-competent virus beyond 10 days that may warrant extending duration of isolation and precautions for up to 20 days after symptom onset; severely immunocompromised patients may produce replication-competent virus beyond 20 days and require additional testing and consultation with infectious diseases specialists and infection control experts.
>
> For adults who never develop symptoms, isolation and other precautions can be discontinued 10 days after the date of their first positive RT-PCR test result for SARS-CoV-2 RNA or 7 days depending upon symptoms. If individuals do not develop symptoms, they need only quarantine for 10 days; if they test negative, that period can be reduced to just one week.

Public health decisions are made based on general safety and economic impacts on the community as a whole. It is understood that a shortened isolation period would allow some infection to spread but would also allow more persons to work and continue activities. If there is a mutation that makes this germ more dangerous, the length of time would again be changed to a longer period for the greater good.

What is the lag time from start of illness to potential death in a seriously ill individual?

Mean time from start of symptoms to death is 12.9 to 19.2 days among those who die.[2] The infection fatality rate is highly variable, among age groups particularly, and this is discussed further in the book. In fact, the purpose of this book is to explain how to minimize finding yourself among this unenviable group.

What is the most important concept to learn about taking appropriate (not over, not under) precautions against SARS-CoV-2?

Understanding the concept of ID_{50} and MID, discussed further in chapter 2, is important for being able to understand why immunizations, masks, and other social engineering can make a difference in controlling the disease. The ID_{50} stand for the infectious dose of a germ that will infect 50 percent of the people exposed to that dose, and MID is the minimum infectious dose that will give an individual an infection. This is the most important concept there is in developing a plan to minimize becoming infected and at the same time maximize normal daily life. The minimum infectious dose of SARS-CoV-2 that will get you ill depends on your age and multiple other conditions. Understanding those conditions will help you understand what chances you can "safely" take, or at least how to greatly minimize your risk.

Can you trust the results of a Covid-19 test?

Only if it is taken at the correct time from exposure and from the correct location of your body, and is the right type of test (discussed in detail in chapter 5). Beware of why there could be false negative and prolonged meaningless positive PCRs. This is the test taken by nasal or buccal swabs and processed by a technique called polymerase chain reaction. Understand that the sensitivity and specificity of a test varies with the percentage positivity of the test in the population. This is a rather difficult concept to understand, so you had better see the full discussion in chapter 5.

How many people are asymptomatic?

Estimates have ranged that between 40 and 80 percent of people are either *asymptomatic* or *pre-symptomatic* when they have the disease. The asymptomatic person never has any symptoms. The pre-symptomatic person has no idea that they are infected and does not feel ill—until suddenly they do feel ill. The lack of availability of testing is complicated by overtesting or inappropriate testing, biasing results. For example, if only symptomatic people are authorized to get tested, the positivity rate will be quite elevated. But if persons are tested too early after contact to show results, or are tested for administrative reasons such as travel, these likely large numbers of negative results will indicate a lower positivity rate. If a certain positivity rate in an area is the benchmark against when schools or other activities may open, the data source will be skewed one way or the other.

Are people contagious when they are asymptomatic or pre-symptomatic?

The game-changing answer is: yes and yes. With most disease, including influenza (and SARS and MERS, the other two deadly coronaviruses in the same species as SARS-CoV-2), people are not contagious prior to becoming ill. It allows doctors to rapidly isolate them from others, without even the need for testing. However, a disease will spread rapidly and widely through a community when those infected do not even know they have it.

How contagious is SARS-CoV-2 virus, and how will the variants change this?

The infectiousness of a disease is called the "R naught," expressed as R_0. In theory this number gives you an idea of how infectious a disease is. The infectiousness of a disease is better expressed by the term "relative infectiousness," or R_e (more detail on both in chapter 3). The population changes and can become less likely to catch the disease (from either surviving infection and gaining natural immunity or receiving vaccine immunity), or become more susceptible (perhaps due to the disease developing a new variant that is more infectious). The issue of how the variants of SARS-CoV-2 might change their infectiousness is discussed in chapter 6. The R naught becomes a critical point of discussion in helping compute the level of immunity required to reach herd immunity. The more contagious a disease, the higher the herd immunity must be.

Can variants cause the vaccines to fail to protect me? Can variants fool tests? Will variants change treatments and how?
Yes, yes, and yes. That is the bad news. It is also possible that variants will develop a weakness we can exploit, and better treat, and that will eventually replace multiple variants with just a few "winners" that can be more easily targeted with vaccines or preventive medication. The main trick is to prevent them from forming in the first place. Variants—their challenges and solutions—are discussed in chapter 6.

CHAPTER 2

THE MINIMAL INFECTIOUS DOSE

The singular most important concept in surviving SARS-CoV-2 is understanding that this disease, like all others, has a minimum infective dose of greater than one particle to get you infected, and it can also be expected that a certain number of the virus particles would get about 50 percent of a group infected.

The understanding of the concept of median infective dose is critical to making a decision about the importance of masks, social distancing, and the use of vaccines. Virtually any logical basis for dealing with the social impacts of mitigating this disease will take advantage of the fact that this disease, like every disease, has a MID_{50} and a minimum infective dose. Many of you will not be familiar with this term. It has not been discussed in any of the "Covid Task Force" presentations.

MID_{50} is prime proof that medicine is not binary—it is not a "yes" or "no" type of business. The MID_{50} refers to the dose of an infectious agent that will cause 50 percent of a group of people to catch a disease. This is why masks and social distancing can both work and fail to work. If you were to get sick from a disease by being exposed to only one germ, almost nothing would protect you. You would have to be in a very protective bubble to prevent a single germ from contacting you. You are contacted by germs all the time—numerous different kinds of germs, even including SARS-CoV-2. The reason you are not sick, not dead, is because your defense against these germs is robust enough to protect you from most of them. When you do get sick, it is because you are exposed to a large enough number of germs of that disease that it overwhelms your immune response.

The purpose of masks, for example, is not to totally prevent the spread of germs (no masks are that efficient), but to decrease the number that are inhaled (or exhaled by someone else) to a low enough number that your body is able to destroy the ones that get through.

Some diseases are so virulent that exposure to even one cell can make you ill. That is a very rare beastie. Studies have been conducted on a number of germs that identify the various MID_{50}s. Most viruses enter the body through the respiratory or the gastrointestinal tracts. It is rather easy to measure the MID_{50} of the ingested infectious dose as you can just have the test subject drink various concentrations.

For diseases that spread through aerosol, the measurement is trickier but can be computed from either epidemiological data or laboratory studies.

All organisms have a minimum infectious dose—the dose required to make a person ill. As can be seen, there is quite a range, with some organisms requiring fewer than ten to make a person ill and others requiring as many as a billion to cause illness.

For example:

Hepatitis A	10–100 virus particles
Norovirus	10–100 virus particles
Rotavirus	10–100 virus particles
Salmonella	6–23 bacteria
Shigella	200 bacteria

Some organisms have been shown to usually require very large amounts to cause illness:

Streptococcus pyogenes	1,000 bacteria
Campylobacter	500–800 bacteria
E. coli	1M–1B bacteria
E. coli O157:H7	10–100 bacteria
Vibrio parahaemolyticus	1,000 bacteria
Vibrio cholera	1,000 bacteria
The O139 serotype	10,000 bacteria
Yersinia enterocolitica	1M–1B bacteria

Note that all of the above diseases are intestinal and come from ingesting germs from food or water.

Various studies have been performed to determine the median infective dose that would infect half the persons subjected to the airborne germs.[1]

Respiratory

Adenovirus—small particle aerosol	6.6 virus particles
RSV strain A2—nasal drops	501 plaque-forming units

Enteric

Rotavirus—oral ingestion	0.9 focus-forming units
Poliovirus—gelatin capsule	1 tissue culture infective dose 50
Norovirus—oral suspension	18 viruses
Chovirus—oral suspension	17 plaque-forming units
Giardia lamblia—oral ingestion	25–100 cysts

This data shows that with the very contagious norovirus, the disease that frequently causes vomiting and diarrhea for cruise ship passengers, maybe one hundred virus particles are required to get an individual sick, but eighteen virus particles have been shown to make 50 percent of those subjected to that dose ill. Some people are more susceptible to the disease, while others are more resistant.

This holds true for any disease. Some individuals will be made ill with a very low number of germs, while others will tolerate a much higher level without getting sick. A certain level will get at least 50 percent of those exposed ill, and there is certainly an ID, or infectious dose, that will get anyone ill.

Why is there a variation in how much virus is required to cause a person to catch a specific illness?
A number of protective factors prevent one virus or even significant doses of some diseases to infect a particular individual.

It could be the method by which the disease penetrates the body and invades cells. In the case of SARS-CoV-2, the spike proteins attach to ace receptors. Young children have fewer ace receptors in their nasal mucosa lining than do older children and adults, and thus may not be as susceptible to the same cloud of virus particles that would infect an older person. In other words, they lack, or have a paucity of, virus receptors. A similar issue regarding a difference in the number of receptors causing different disease rates is noted regarding norovirus in the table above. Twenty percent of Europeans are not susceptible to that disease as they do not genetically produce large numbers of the viral receptor in their nasal or respiratory tract.[2]

A person might sneeze and dislodge so many virus particles that they effectively "clean out" enough to mechanically clear themselves. The mechanical "cleansing" is also noted in some gastrointestinal diseases that can cause vomiting or diarrhea. This is partially why the MID_{50} of some *E. coli* and *Yersinia enterocolitica* are so high, as noted in the above table. When it comes to upper respiratory illness, the sneezing and coughing serves two almost divergent purposes: It rids the body of many germs it then does not have to fight, and, from the germs' point of view, it helps them spread to others.

Partial or full immunity is a major factor why one individual can withstand larger doses of a particular germ than another person. But full immunity is a misnomer. There is no such thing. Even a strong immunity to a particular disease can be overwhelmed by a large enough inoculum to cause an individual to fall ill. Thus, social distancing, efforts such as appropriate air flow control and avoiding contaminated surfaces, and masks serve primarily to reduce the number of virus particles entering a person's body (and leaving another person in the case of masks) to the point that the number of germs received is below the minimum infectious dose for that individual.

CHAPTER 3

WHAT IS THE R NAUGHT FOR SARS-COV-2 AND WHAT ARE THE IMPLICATIONS?

The R naught (R_o), or basic reproduction number, indicates how infectious a pathogen is by estimating the average number of people who will contract a disease from one person with that disease. A R_o less than 1 means a disease will not become an epidemic, as it will slowly dwindle in number of cases with fewer and fewer people catching it from a first case. A higher R_o indicates a greater number of individuals will be infected from a single infected individual.

R_o (basic reproduction number) of diseases

A measure of how many people each sick person will infect on average

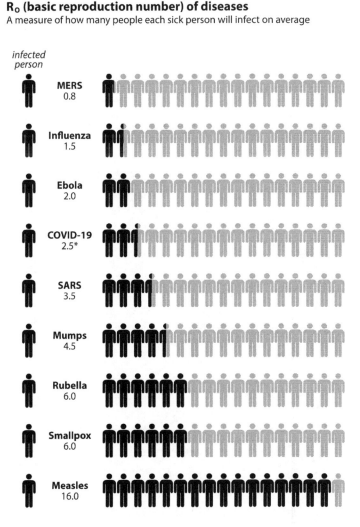

This number may change as we learn more about this new disease

This number is calculated on the exposure to persons naïve to the disease with no immunity from natural disease or immunization and no social engineering such as distancing, washing, or masking being effectively used to prevent the disease spread.

As an example, measles is extremely infectious with an R_0 typically between 12 and 18, which works out to a herd-immunity threshold requirement of 92 to 94 percent of the population.

When the virus that causes Covid-19 was first evaluated, the R_0 was estimated to be from 2.2 to 5.8. That range is hotly contested, as it influences the percentage of a population that needs to be immune to reach herd immunity. It would seem possible to set a goal to achieve herd immunity, through a combination of natural disease and immunization, at 54 percent, if the R_0 is 2.2, but an R_0 of 5.8 would require a herd immunity of 83 percent, probably unachievable. So the R_0 of 2.2 that is usually claimed for this disease by government officials may be purposely low so that the herd immunity goal will seem more approachable.

The higher estimates for R_0 of up to 5.8 would mean herd immunity could not be achieved without almost 100 percent acceptance of immunization—a very unlikely scenario. In fact, as mutation variants become more widespread, the efficiency of available vaccines will probably not be high enough to form herd immunity that will be protective. That's a tragic thought, because then the only thing left is social distancing, masks, etc.

Here are three stories from the *New York Times* that illustrate the dangers of SARS-CoV-2 with an R_0 that varies, depending on the social event, from probably 2.2 to 5.8:[1]

1. In Manassas, Virginia, Christine Pabico had spent months protecting her 73-year-old father, who lived with her along with his wife, from being exposed to the virus. But after a nine-person family get-together, Ms. Pabico's sister developed a fever. She had been exposed, unknowingly, to the virus the day before Thanksgiving, and it spread rapidly throughout the home.

    Eventually her father was admitted to the hospital. And on the day it became clear he would not make it, hospital staff

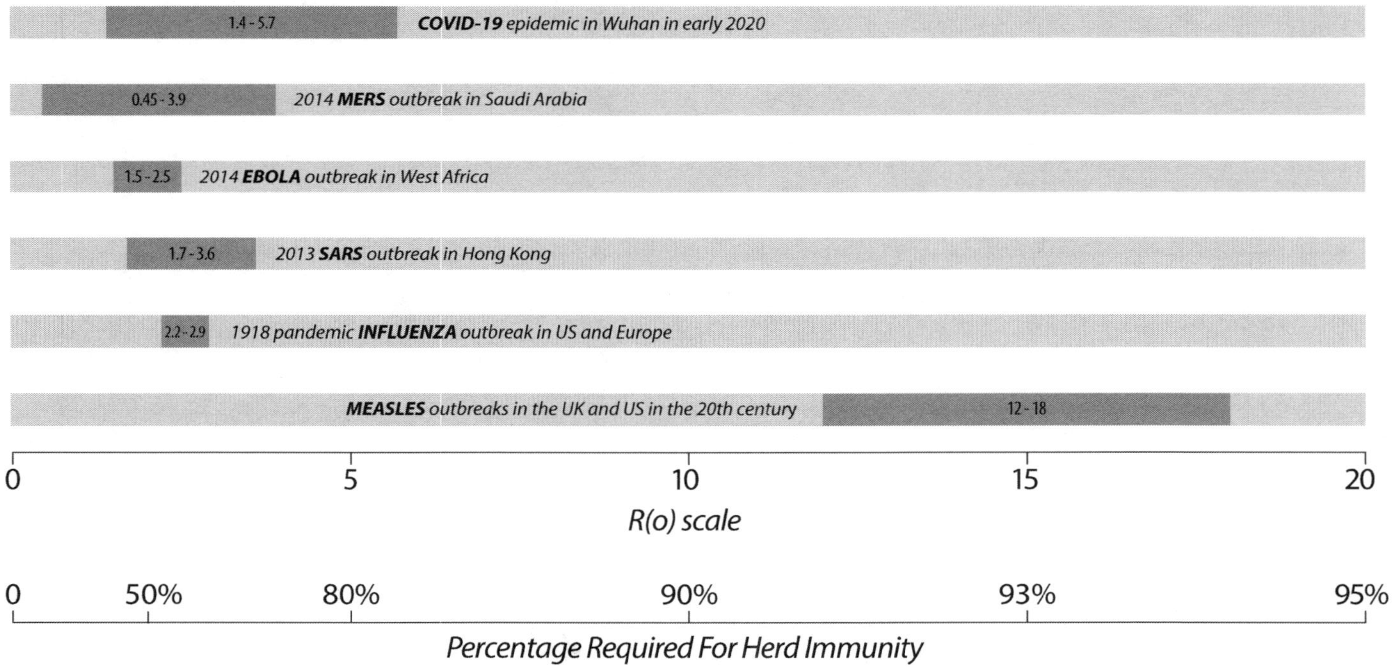

COVID-19 epidemic in Wuhan in early 2020
1.4 - 5.7

2014 MERS outbreak in Saudi Arabia
0.45 - 3.9

2014 EBOLA outbreak in West Africa
1.5 - 2.5

2013 SARS outbreak in Hong Kong
1.7 - 3.6

1918 pandemic INFLUENZA outbreak in US and Europe
2.2 - 2.9

MEASLES outbreaks in the UK and US in the 20th century
12 - 18

0	5	10	15	20

R(o) scale

0	50%	80%	90%	93%	95%

Percentage Required For Herd Immunity

As can be seen by the above illustration, a very slight increase of the R naught (R_o) above 2 requires a much larger herd immunity to protect the population from disease. The formula is Herd Immunity=$1/R_o$. Linear R_o.

SCALE AND HERD IMMUNITY DIAGRAM COURTESY DAVID R. SCOTT

allowed his family to join him to say goodbye. For his final request, he asked that they bring him his favorite brand of coffee ice cream, and Philippine adobo with rice.

2. In Texas, Danny Cooke, 62, and his family decided to play it safe on Thanksgiving in Fort Worth. He and his wife hosted an intimate dinner with Mr. Cooke's daughter, her husband, and their two children. They opened all the windows and let the Texas air flow through the nouse.

But by the weekend, Mr. Cooke's daughter, Amanda Ayala, a pediatric nurse, started to show symptoms of Covid-19. She tested positive, and several days later so did Mr. Cooke and his wife.

"We kind of thought we were OK," Mr. Cooke said. "But obviously, that was the wrong thing to do."

Mr. Cooke's wife and daughter have both since recovered. But more than three weeks later, he is still struggling with a fever and a cough. On Thursday, Ms. Ayala went to her father's home to check his blood pressure and oxygen levels. She blames herself for getting him sick.

"It weighs on me," she said. "I'm just hoping for it to pass."

Mr. Cooke had been working in-person during the pandemic at Lockheed Martin. He has come into contact with many people at work. But it was at home, at a holiday gathering of six, where he believes he caught the virus.

"Of course, as my wife keeps telling me, 'You can't let this kill you, because your daughter will never forgive herself,' he said."

3. Oscar Gutierrez, 36, a city councilman in Santa Barbara's Westside, urged his mother not to attend a small Thanksgiving dinner with relatives. He lives with his 70-year-old mother and his girlfriend, and he had been taking the precautions seriously, attending council meetings virtually for months from his living room. He and his girlfriend celebrated Thanksgiving at home. But his mother decided to go to the dinner.

"She kind of just got overtaken by the pandemic fatigue, and she wanted to see her relatives and so she went out," Mr. Gutierrez said. "They had their dinner outside. They kept it to less than three households and they were only there for a couple hours. But that's all it took."

Days later, one of the relatives started to feel sick, so he and his mother got tested. They were both infected.

"I was pretty upset," he said. "I lost my temper a little bit. I've spent over ten months not getting it, and then all it took was one dinner and I got it."

Even with an R_0 of 2.2 to 5.8, we can see from our experience with SARS-CoV-2 that the spread in small groups can be impressive, as the above stories illustrate. Social events involving the production of "jets" of aerosols, as in singing or shouting, have produced even more impressive spreads.

A report hit the news media in March 2020 with an early warning of the rather high R_0 that SARS-CoV-2 had.

Skagit County, Washington, had not reported any cases of Covid-19, schools and businesses remained open, and prohibitions on large gatherings had not yet been announced. On March 6, Adam Burdick, the choir's conductor, informed the 121 members in an email that amid the "stress and strain of concerns about the virus," practice would proceed as scheduled at Mount Vernon Presbyterian Church.

"I'm planning on being there this Tuesday, March 10, and hoping many of you will be, too," he wrote.

Sixty singers showed up, and a greeter offered hand sanitizer at the door. Members refrained from the usual hugs and handshakes.

"It seemed like a normal rehearsal, except that choirs are huggy places," Burdick recalled. "We were making music and trying to keep a certain distance between each other."

After two and a half hours, the singers parted ways at 9 p.m.

Nearly three weeks later, forty-five choir members had been diagnosed with Covid-19 or were ill with the symptoms, three were hospitalized, and two were dead.

That event is typical of a super-spreader. It is not that the germ has become more dangerous or that a variant has developed; rather, it is the formation of jets of aerosol in a closed space that effectively raises the R naught, or more precisely, the R effective factor (R_e). The germ with the same R naught, in other words, varies in its effective infectiousness by the behavior and the level of immunity of the population to which it is being exposed.

CHAPTER 4

HERD IMMUNITY

The end of a pandemic is when the population reaches herd immunity, caused either by enough people reaching immune status from infection or immunization, or by unfortunately dying off. If the R naught or, more accurately, the R_e infection factor drops below 1 from increased immunity, the disease will slowly die out.

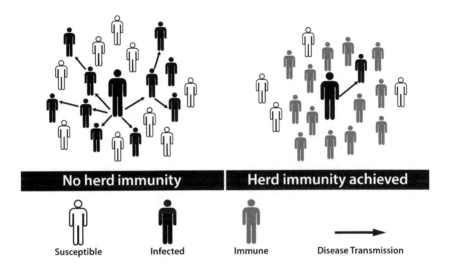

No herd immunity	Herd immunity achieved

Susceptible Infected Immune Disease Transmission

Many childhood diseases with decreased immunization rates have resulted in a loss of herd immunity. If the percentage of a group loses herd immunity (drops below the herd immunity threshold), a single case can spread like wildfire through the entire group, even infecting those who have some immunity. An overwhelming number of germs results during infection outbreaks. Depending on how virulent the germ is and how easily it spreads, a stronger level of immunity must be present to prevent this "wildfire" spread. The level of immunity a group must have to prevent disease spread is called the "herd immunity."

It is interesting that some of the most dangerous diseases have a relatively low herd immunity required for group protection from disease acceleration. Ebola has a high case-fatality rate of 60 to 90 percent in the case of the Zaire strain and 40 to 60 percent in the Sudan variety. Its herd immunity is low because its method of spread requires direct contact.

On the other hand, for a large potential number of deaths on the planet, it is hard to beat the danger of influenza. An aggressive strain of influenza could reach a mortality rate of 2.5 percent, as the disease spreads easily among nonimmune persons. When virtually everyone catches it (unlike Ebola, which no one should catch with simple body fluid precautions), the death toll can be astounding.

Herd immunity for rabies in wild dogs is reached when 40 percent of the dog population is immunized against rabies. Again, like Ebola, rabies is an extremely dangerous disease with almost 100 percent mortality. Yet the herd immunity for dogs is low since it requires actual biting for it to spread.

Airborne diseases can spread easily, so the herd immunity to prevent them exploding in a population is high.

	Transmission	Herd Immunity Required	R_0—The R Naught Reproduction Number
Measles	Airborne	92–95%	12–18
Pertussis (whooping cough)	Airborne droplet	92–94%	5.5
Diphtheria	Saliva	83–86%	1.7–4.3
Rubella	Airborne droplet	83–86%	6–7
Smallpox	Airborne droplet	80–86%	3.5–6
Polio	Fecal–oral route	80–86%	5–7
Mumps	Airborne droplet	75–86%	10–12
SARS	Airborne droplet	60–80%	0.19–1.1
SARS-CoV-2	Aerosol	80–90%	2.1–5.8
MERS	Airborne droplet	unknown	0.3–0.8
Ebola	Bodily fluids direct contact	33–60%	1.5–1.9
Influenza	Airborne droplet	33–44%	1.1–1.6

Sometimes herd immunity does not protect you from a disease—tetanus, for example, as you catch this directly from spores via skin punctures and not from another person.

An unsuspecting release of a bioterrorism weapon may require the use of treatment, if available, for curative or supportive care. But in case of significant threat, the best protection is immunization. This is also true for the naturally occurring diseases.

CHAPTER 5

WHAT ARE THE DIFFERENT TESTS FOR COVID-19 AND CAN I TRUST THE RESULTS?

WHAT TYPES OF TESTS ARE COMMONLY USED TO DETECT SARS-COV-2?

There are four major types of tests for SARS-CoV-2 disease. Each test has its own sensitivity and specificity established to indicate its accuracy. Of course, there are a number of manufacturers, and their tests have individual levels of specificity and sensitivity for each type of test.

PCR Testing

The most common test is a molecular test that will directly test for the virus particle—all of which are considered nucleic acid amplification tests. Of the various types of these tests, the most sensitive and specific is the Reverse Transcription Polymerase Chain Reaction or RT-PCR, commonly referred to as a "PCR test." This is performed either as a swab deep in the nose, a swab at the end of the nose (usually performed as a dab into each nostril), or from a mouth swab or saliva spit test. These tests cannot tell if the virus particle is infective, only that it is there. This is an important distinction. For these tests to be accurate, the timing is critical. As can be seen from the illustrations below, a person can be exposed and actively incubating the disease, perhaps for 4 to 6 days, even being contagious to others, yet not feel sick themselves. Early in that period not enough virus particles are there to be picked up by a PCR test. The test will be negative, not because the test in inaccurate, but because it was taken at the wrong time. The virus had not yet multiplied to the point where it could be collected. The other caution is that this test may stay positive for weeks (even 83 days) after symptom onset—long after the person is no longer infective. These people are just shedding inactive virus particles.

Another more available molecular test is the CRISPR-based test, which also detects nucleic acid from the virus ribonucleic acid (RNA). CRISPR stands for "clustered regularly interspaced short palindromic repeats" and uses a powerful genetic-editing technology that cuts into the viral gene. As more tests are produced, they may be available at a lower cost and be more accurate than the PCR test. Like the PCR, the CRISPR-based test will not be able to tell if the virus is infectious or just an inactive particle. It also will have the same limitation of requiring that the test be performed at the correct time. Expect it to be most accurate about 2 days before the person becomes ill (approximately 4 days after contact) and remain accurate for about 10 days after symptom onset. It also will continue to be positive long after active infectious particles are no longer there, just inactive virus bits and pieces.

Antigen Testing

An antigen test is also performed as a deep nasal swab, not so deep nasal swab, throat swab, or saliva spit test. This test detects proteins produced by the virus. There are twenty-nine proteins that make up the SARS-CoV-2 virus. Much of the work being done on test and vaccine development is against the proteins making the S spike protein (several types of them) and the capsule substance called nucleocapsid phosphoprotein N.

As many of the currently circulating coronaviruses in the United States (there are four other types present besides SARS-CoV-2) have similar N proteins, these can give false positive results to some antigen tests. The better antigen tests look for specific parts of the S protein unique to SARS-CoV-2. The most accurate part of this S protein, the part not shared by the other coronaviruses, is a part called the RBD, the receptor binding domain. The other proteins present are the nucleocapsid (N) protein, the envelope (E) protein, and the membrane (M) protein—all of which are antigens.

The antigen tests will most likely be accurate from about 2 days before symptoms develop (4 days after exposure) to days after symptom development.

Antibody Testing

Your body starts making antibodies called IgA, IgM, and IgG within one to two weeks of the onset of infection. These antibodies will last for weeks, at least eight, and may be detectable for much longer. These are the humoral antibodies as opposed to the cell-mediated immune response consisting of B-cell and T-cells, which may well last a lifetime.

CORONAVIRUS PROTEINS

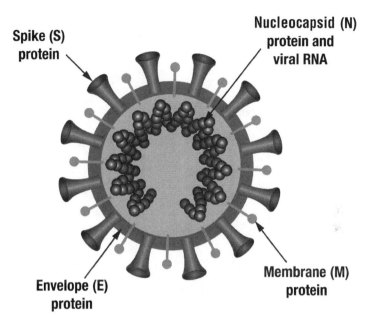

The various components of the coronavirus act as antigens that cause the body to produce antibodies. They are also the machinery that protects the virus and enables it to attach to a cell and reproduce itself. Tests are designed to detect the RNA, the N nucleocapsid protein, the S glycoprotein, the E protein, the M protein, and the underlying lipid bilayer membrane, among other structures. Antibody tests are designed to identify the specific antibodies your body makes to defend against these viral antigen proteins.

Testing for the appropriate B-cells and T-cells is exceedingly difficult and will not be available as routine tests, but testing is an important research tool to determine how long persons will remain immune due to natural disease or immunizations.

Your bone marrow is continuously producing stem cells that then differentiate into all the various types of blood cells, including various white cells and your red blood cells. One type of white blood cell is the lymphocyte—of which there are two types: B cells and T cells. The B cells produce the antibodies that directly destroy foreign

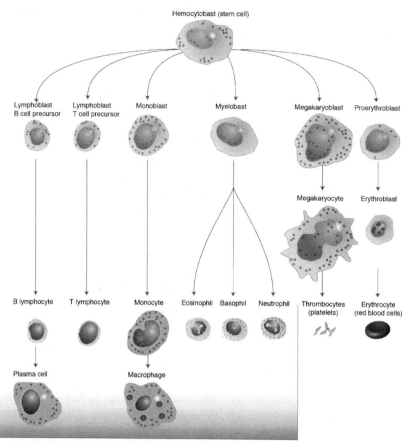

Lymphocytes - white blood cells

The differentiation of cells from stem cells produced in the body. While many of these cells are involved in defending the body from parasites, bacteria, and viruses, the most important response for long-term immunity is made via the B and T lymphocytes.

ILLUSTRATION COURTESY NATIONAL HUMAN GENOME RESEARCH INSTITUTE, WWW.GENOME.GOV.

invaders such as bacteria, viruses, and parasites, and they accomplish this by forming plasma cells to secrete specific antibodies and, with the help of T cells, activate various inflammation pathways, which also aid in destroying invaders. It is sometimes an overreaction of the inflammation process that causes some of the harm during Covid-19 infections. Many of the treatments for this disease are geared to decreasing the inflammatory response, while some treatments are geared toward killing the virus itself.

The value of testing for antibodies is to demonstrate that a person has had a particular disease and to help determine if they are immune.

Antibody testing can usually be done as a rapid point-of-care test. This means it can be done in a clinic office and with home test kits, providing the results in just a few minutes. But note that the best time to obtain an accurate test result will be about 10 days to eight weeks after onset of symptoms. As the test will be dependent upon which antibody it is testing for, it may give a false positive to a recent exposure to one of the other more harmless coronaviruses. A positive test means you have had the disease in the last 10 days to perhaps six months ago and that you are possibly immune.

Some B cells are specific cells that remember the same pathogen for faster antibody production in future infections. A negative test for an antibody does not mean that you are not immune, as the majority of your immunity is provided by these specific B cells and T cells for the long haul. Both from immunizations and natural disease, this cell-mediated immunity may last for many years, perhaps a lifetime.

VIRUS CULTURE

A viable virus culture means that the virus that was tested was able to reproduce when placed into experimental laboratory cells. This is the proof that the virus tested was contagious. Nasal swabs for the PCR test only identify that virus particles were found, not that the virus was capable of infection. You may remain positive for viral particles for an average of 17 days (maximum tested so far has been 83 days), while most people are probably not contagious after 10 days from onset of symptoms.

The appropriate location for taking the test changes as the virus moves through the system—starting at the nose, then working its way deeper to the nasal pharynx, and finally into the lungs. Nasal secretions for PCR may remain positive for an average of 17 days as mentioned above, but they may become negative long before. The actual infection is moving deeper as it continues, so even nasal swab PCR tests are frequently negative when a person is dying of severe lung infection, while they may remain falsely positive when the person is immune and no longer shedding contagious virus particles (only nonviable virus particles). Properly performed, the virus culture proves infection is present.

GENOMIC SEQUENCING

The SARS-CoV-2 virus was first detected in China in December (perhaps October) 2019. While the Chinese were very selective and secretive about the significance of this illness, thus catching the world off-guard, they did rapidly perform full genome sequencing, releasing this information on January 10, 2020. Genomic sequencing is the full, detailed description of the RNA that makes the virus unique. RNA consists of pairs of nucleotides, as does the double-stranded DNA that makes up our cells. RNA uses a slightly different nucleotide code than DNA and, like this virus, is virtually always in a single strand. (Nothing in nature is, of course, always.)

It was the Chinese genome sequencing that discovered that this new illness was a coronavirus, and that it was related to SARS, MERS, and the other four circulating, less harmful coronavirus colds. It was this sequencing that allowed scientists to discern which part of the virus genome or sequence was responsible for enabling various components of the new virus to command an infected cell to reproduce thousands of copies. Specific parts of the genome sequence cause it to make the spike proteins, the nucleocapsid, envelope, and membrane proteins, and the various other components of the virus.

As we see mutations in the spike protein, they may reduce, but not obliterate, the recognition of the virus by antibodies. This is because the immune system will recognize more than a single region of the spike protein. The spike protein is made up of 1,273 amino acids, and changes in one or a few of its amino acids is usually not enough to stop recognition of the whole protein.

But the test—genomic sequencing—is the test necessary to identify when these mutations appear, how fast they spread, and if they cause more or even less severe illness, enable resistance to various vaccines or treatments, or attack various age groups differently.

Compared to Europe and some Asian countries, the United States is very behind in using genome sequencing testing for the public health issues noted above. But this process is of necessity speeding up and is being accelerated worldwide. There is now global collaboration to collect and analyze SARS-CoV-2 sequence data. There are hundreds of thousands of complete SARS-CoV-2 genomes available, with this number increasing daily. To see the very latest tables and maps of the appearance of various mutations of this virus, go to www.coronacov19.com.

To access the database of variant mutations appearing in the United States, go to www.cdc.gov and search for the term "Variant Proportions in the U.S." A biweekly chart shows the rapid increase of variants like the British (Kent or B.1.1.7), the South African (B.1.352), the Brazilan (P.1), and many US-originated variants. Also noted is the percentage of variant by state derived from the (so far) low amount of genomic testing performed in the United States. The chart is updated every two weeks.

TESTING ACCURACY

The major factors that affect how accurate a test will be are as follows:

1. *The type of test must be performed at the right time from exposure to the illness through recovery.*

   This is illustrated below. As can be seen by the diagram, when testing for the virus by PCR, one can expect the particle to not be detectable for perhaps 5 days from the time of infection. Thus, an initial negative test can (in fact will) be a false negative. Once beyond the 10-day period, the nasal swab PCR for virus particles will still show positive, but by then the particles are not viable and so a positive test does not mean (necessarily) that the person is still infectious—and they may by then not even be clinically ill. Asymptomatic carriers will never be ill but will show a positive PCR test within a 5- to 10-day period in which they will be contagious, and positive after that, when they will probably not be contagious.

SARS-CoV-2 Viral Load and Appropriate Testing

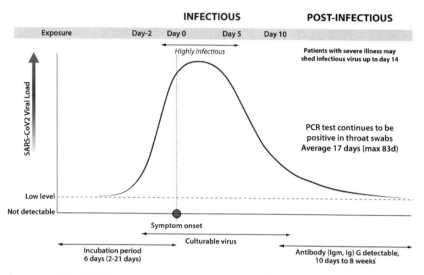

As the above illustration indicates, for some days after contact with the disease, there is an exceptionally low viral load, or virus count, in the patient. About 4 days after contact with the disease, and about 2 days before the person becomes ill, the virus load rises and stays high until about 10 days after the illness has started. The typical ill person can be contagious for 2 to maybe 4 days before developing symptoms and may remain contagious for 14 days due to infectious virus shedding during that time. But by day 10 of onset of infection, most people are not shedding infectious virus. They may shed nonviable virus particles; that is, virus particles that can be measured by PCR testing, but which are not contagious. Antibodies (IgM, IgG) are detectable starting within 10 days and strong for usually six to eight weeks.

2. *The test must be obtained from the correct part of the anatomy.* Infectious viral particles will start showing up where the disease starts—in the nose. They then descend into the pharynx and then into the lungs. Thus, a PCR test is able to show these particles at different time frames of the illness.

3. *The sample must be stored and transported to the lab correctly.* Some samples, such as those taken for antigen tests, must be processed within 1½ hours to be accurate. Others require specific transport solutions, and still others must be sent dry. Transport temperatures also can be critical for a specific specimen.

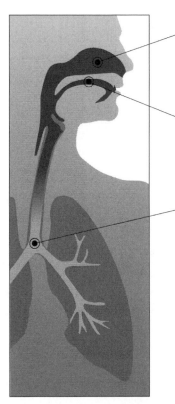

Nasal swab – for PCR test – fewer viral particles will be found in the outer nares and for a shorter time than in the deep nasal-pharyngeal region.

Saliva swab and spit test – for antigen and PCR testing – most accurate 2 days before to 7 days after onset of symptoms.

Bronchial lavage – for PCR, antigen and live viral testing – only if the patient has pneumonia and/or intubation. These will be positive when the PCS nares test might be negative.

Finger blood test – for antibodies – most accurate 2 weeks to 8 weeks after symptoms.

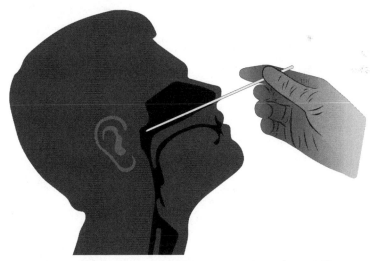

The dreaded "deep" nasal-pharyngeal swab, correctly performed. This location will yield the most accurate results for PCR tests from approximately 2 days before symptoms to 10 days afterward. This location can remain positive longer than throat swabs, but these are probably nonviable virus fragments and likely do not indicate virus that can infect others after that time.

4. *The lab must not contaminate the sample (easily done during a PCR test).*

PCR tests are magnifying a small segment of the RNA particle. The slightest microscopic amount in, for example, the laboratory lab bench protection hood, can cause false positives, as several national sports teams found out, causing them to cancel games and isolate players, at least temporarily, until the confirmation tests disproved the false result.

5. *The physician must know how to interpret the test.*

Interpretation will depend on the physician knowing the time of exposure and the anatomical location of the specimen collection as discussed above, and the sensitivity and specificity as discussed below.

6. *The test will have a certain sensitivity and specificity that significantly affects the result's accuracy depending on the percentage of people infected with the disease.*

Sensitivity and specificity seem easy to understand but can be tricky to interpret. The easiest way to think of this is to consider a car that has a burglar alarm. If the alarm is very sensitive, it will go off whenever a robber tries to steal it. But if it is too sensitive, it will also go off falsely when somebody just walks by. Specificity relates to the test identifying the correct illness and not a similar one; in other words, it correctly identifies the burglar from an innocent passerby. The positive predictive value is the description of "how often is the test true?"

As you can see from the following diagram, the number of false positive and false negative test results is influenced greatly by the amount of disease that is active in the community. If there is a lot of disease present in a community, the chance of a positive test being correct is high (if correctly sampled both by location and time from start of exposure). When the disease is extremely high in a community, the chance of a properly obtained, negative test being a false negative becomes more likely.

In other words, when a disease is active in a community, a positive test is usually true and a negative is possibly inaccurate.

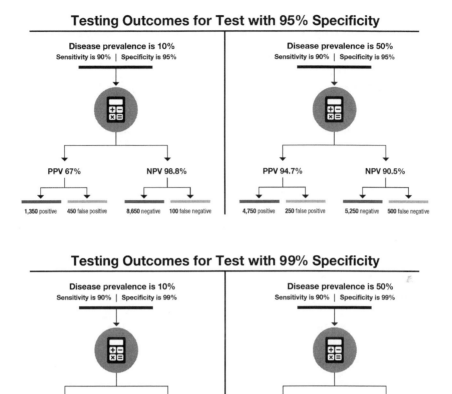

Testing Outcomes for Test with 95% Specificity

Disease prevalence is 10%
Sensitivity is 90% | Specificity is 95%

PPV 67%   NPV 98.8%

1,350 positive   450 false positive   8,650 negative   100 false negative

Disease prevalence is 50%
Sensitivity is 90% | Specificity is 95%

PPV 94.7%   NPV 90.5%

4,750 positive   250 false positive   5,250 negative   500 false negative

Testing Outcomes for Test with 99% Specificity

Disease prevalence is 10%
Sensitivity is 90% | Specificity is 99%

PPV 90.9%   NPV 98.9%

990 positive   90 false positive   9,010 negative   100 false negative

Disease prevalence is 50%
Sensitivity is 90% | Specificity is 99%

PPV 98.9%   NPV 90.8%

4,550 positive   50 false positive   5,450 negative   500 false negative

Obtaining the correct test at the correct time is essential. As the germs congregate at different parts of the body (nose, throat, lungs), in greater concentrations at different periods of time from the start of incubation, the sample site and timing of acquisition are both important for accuracy. Taking the sample too soon or too late can give false results.

What do you do if the test is negative, but you are sick with Covid-19 symptoms?

Some of the rapid tests that look at antigens may be fooled by a variant. Also, as seen in the discussion on testing accuracy, there may be false negative tests even under the best of circumstances. In this situation it is best to have a repeat test, perhaps using a different technique (rather than an antigen test, perhaps a PCR test). In medical parlance this is called orthogonal testing. It is basically any method of testing—or test kit, which could be the same type of test—that provides a different sensitivity or specificity.

If you are ill, even with a negative test:

- Treat yourself as if you do have Covid-19. Rest and use acetaminophen for fever and aches. Severe joint pain might respond better to a nonsteroidal anti-inflammatory such as ibuprofen.
- Follow your fever course with a good thermometer.
- Obtain a pulse oximeter and follow your percentage blood-oxygen level. If it drops below 94 percent and you are feeling weak and ill, go to the hospital. If it drops below 90 percent, you are in trouble and must go immediately to the hospital.

I cannot overemphasize the importance of rest and adequate hydration. If you have risk factors for complications from this illness (age, obesity, diabetes, high blood pressure, etc.) call your local hospital, as you may qualify for infusion of antibodies (either monoclonal or hopefully polyclonal) and other antiviral therapy early in the disease course. Self-treating with other modalities such as vitamin D, zinc, and so on, is not a substitute for reaching out for the latest version of antiviral therapy that has been developed by modern science.

This is a disease that can progress very gradually. It might incubate with a mild onset and then suddenly become explosive in its behavior. If you have appropriate symptoms, particularly aching, malaise, and fever, even with a negative test, take care of yourself and reach out for help if your condition seems to worsen.

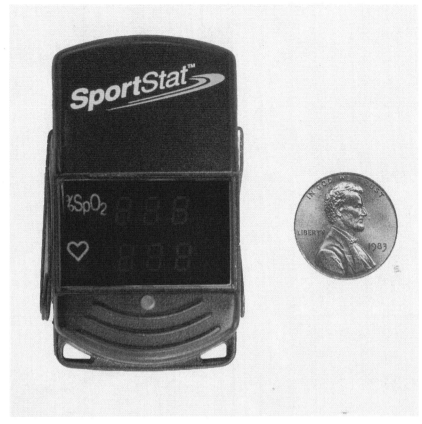

Pulse oximeters are inexpensive (usually below $40) and are in good supply during this late pandemic period.

IMAGE COURTESY DAVID R. SCOTT

CHAPTER 6
MUTATIONS

How do mutations form?

What is a convergent or a selective mutation?

How dangerous are SARS-CoV-2 mutations and will they affect vaccines, treatment, and prevention?

When this nonliving particle, the SARS-CoV-2 virus, floats along and encounters a proper host cell by chance, it has several things its "simple" structure must accomplish. First, it has to avoid being destroyed by the environment or the immune system of the cell it is "attacking." For the attack to work it must attach to the cell, penetrate the cell's protective coating, then be able to grab the machinery of the cell and make multiple copies of itself. Finally, it must burst out of the cell in as many copies as it can make before the cell disintegrates and becomes useless. Then, it either must spread to other cells in the same person or be coughed, sneezed, or otherwise breathed out of that person to float out and somehow get into another human or appropriate animal.

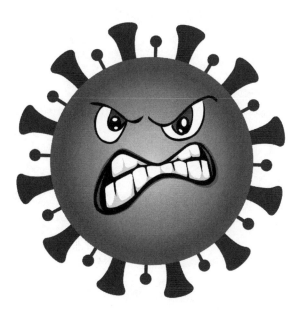

Viruses are "obligate parasites"; to function they must infect a host cell:

- They neither take in nutrients, nor expel waste
- They don't use or expend energy
- They don't grow
- They don't use oxygen
- They don't move on their own
- They can evolve only inside a host cell
- They cannot reproduce on their own

Mutations are not done with cleverness or intelligence. They are accidental and most of the time either mean nothing or even cause the "new, accidentally flawed" copy to become useless. But occasionally one has some advantage in any of the steps mentioned in the paragraph above. Then trouble can really start. The more people who are infected with millions of these virus particles, the more untold trillions of them are being reproduced in those humans. These humans may have no symptoms, but each person infected is an incubator. And all these incubators are the potential incubator where a nasty mutation, one that becomes more infectious, or more lethal, or more resistant to treatment or vaccines, can develop. The need to decrease the number of infected individuals should seem obvious. The more people who are infected, the greater the chance of a nasty mutation forming. So it is no wonder that the United States, with its massive number of infections, would be the ideal place for the most mutations to eventually form—and to probably become the initial home of the very worst.

As indicated in the following figure on page 51, this virus consists of several main types of proteins. Each of these proteins has specific subparts, sometimes with important structural or other functions. Mutations can occur spontaneously at any place in the whole complex system. The mutation is a copying error made from the RNA strand when the hijacked host cell is forced to replicate it. RNA consists of paired nucleotides that inform various messenger RNAs which amino acids to hook together to form the proteins and other structures required to support the new copy of itself. The RNA is replicating itself using energy and components of the host cell. During the event, while the new copy of the virus is being replicated, is the point that an error might be made if it puts the wrong nucleotide into the chain. By definition you have a viable mutation if this little beast survives and is able to function.

When a mutation develops, it can be traced as a lineage. If a group of this virus shares an inherited set of distinctive mutations, especially if it becomes dominant due to its increased infectiousness, it is called a variant. Variants that do not exhibit specifically different characteristics will exist but not be recognized without genome testing (sequencing).

If a lineage develops enough mutations that it exhibits clear clinical differences, it becomes designated as a strain. SARS-CoV-2 is a strain of the SARS virus, a virus species that has been evolving in bats for a long time. There are four common cold types of SARS virus in the United States that are strains as well. The most dangerous SARS strains to date for humans have been the SARS and MERS infections. SARS (Severe Acute Respiratory Syndrome) was discovered in China in 2003 and spread to two dozen countries but was eradicated with no cases reported since 2004. It was eradicated by strong case identification and quarantine. The disease was vicious, with a high case fatality ratio of 10 percent, so it was taken very seriously. Also, it spread mainly by droplet rather than aerosol and only by symptomatic people. Globally 774 people died. MERS, caused by the Middle East respiratory-related coronavirus, was even deadlier with a case fatality rate of 35 percent. Its host animal is the camel, and the potential for spread into humans continues.

SARS-CoV-2 did not come from SARS-1. The leap to human host from bats (probably a leap made ten to fifteen years ago into another animal intermediary) by both SARS-CoV-1 and SARS-CoV-2 is an independent event that can be determined by their genetic structure.

Convergent mutations are mutations that occur in different lines independently. They are probably of benefit, or at least not harmful, when they form and are maintained in the new line.

The genome, the RNA forming the virus genetic material, has 29,764 nucleotide pairs made of four different nucleic acid bases. The four bases are adenine, guanine, cytosine, and uracil. Proteins are made from amino acids. There are twenty naturally occurring amino acids. A strip of three nucleic acids paired together can identify one amino acid. A long strip of these paired amino acids will be able to code for the individual proteins that it wants to attract into a structure. Science has worked out in great detail how this genetic information is utilized for this attraction and how the assembly process works.

Currently, most Covid-19 vaccines target the spike proteins whose job is the attachment to the victim cell it plans to invade. Mutations may reduce vaccine efficacy directed against the spike protein but hopefully will not obliterate their effects. This is because the immune responses they induce target more than a single part of the spike protein. Some vaccines developed, such as inactivated virus vaccines, target an even greater array of viral proteins, inducing several protective immune responses. This instills redundancy in the protective immune responses in case the virus mutates a different structure.

It is still possible that haphazard mutations would accidentally bypass these immune responses by producing a protein structure that replaces the one the immune response has learned to attack. It is a war being waged between a random accidental mutation enabled by millions of human incubators increasing the mathematical chance that such a random accident might happen, and a human immune system trying to protect itself as the attacking virus keeps throwing a new defense into the mix. All are by accident due to these spontaneous mutations from the millions of incubators.

Some of the mutations that different virus variants have, which have been advantageous, are identical—mutations that have arisen spontaneously and not inherited from one lineage. This is known as a convergent evolution, a phenomenon described by Charles Darwin in the mid-1800s in a variety of animals and plants. Different species can develop a body part, like a fin for swimming and, whether it was on a mammal or a fish, it ends up serving the same useful function. Convergent mutations may not serve a useful purpose for the virus, but they can be discovered when we perform genomic sequencing. At times we note a virus mutation variant that seems to have an advantage, perhaps spreading more easily or being more harmful. We may see several variants sharing this advantageous gene but can tell they developed independently, meaning the new, improved gene was not inherited but had developed convergently by luck. (Bad for us, good for it.)

There is a worse scenario where a variant mutation forms due to selective pressure from treatments we use against the virus. Preventions such as immunization or other medications to prevent SARS-CoV-2, or treatments for it once it is caught (medications or manufactured monoclonal or polyclonal antibodies, for instance), will bring a selective pressure on the disease. This means that when a mutation arises that just happens to be resistant to the prevention or treatment, it can become the predominant form of the virus as the treatment or prevention wipes out its competitors, leaving it increasingly dominant and now even more dangerous.

Mutations can occur in various parts of the virus, including various parts of the spike (S) protein, the nucleocapsid (N) protein, the envelope (E) protein, and the membrane (M) protein.

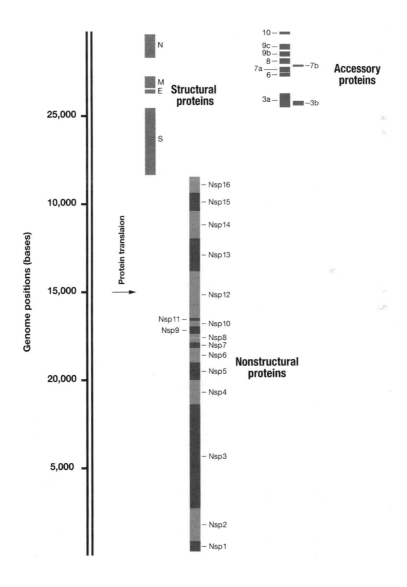

The SARS-CoV-2 structure is composed of 29,903 nucleotides that form a single-strand RNA genome coding the virus to manufacture 29 proteins that have different structures and functions. The virus attaches to cells via its S (spike) protein. The other proteins are essential enzymes required for cell penetration, reproduction, escape, and even defense. The precise functions of many of these proteins are known, but most are a mystery. Once their function is identified, this can enable us to figure out a treatment or prevention targeting that function.

Could the SARS-CoV-2 be an accidental release from a research lab in China or was it a naturally occurring mutation?
A single-strand RNA mutates very easily. With millions of persons infected, mutations are occurring all the time. This particular virus, SARS-CoV-2, whether it came from a lab or animal crossover to humans, once it gains traction in the human population into the millions, it will unquestionably mutate numerous times.

It is important to know that the virus is not a living thing. It cannot just mutate on its own. It *must* be inside a cell it has infected, and only then can it command the cell to reproduce itself. It is during that process that "mistakes" can be made, when the new virus particles are being created. Most of these mistakes are not usable. They do not leave the infected cell because they are unable to, or they cannot infect other cells, or the animal in which they are reproducing dies and they are cremated or buried with it to simply decompose with their victim. Some *are* potentially more infectious (would have a higher R naught) or are more lethal. But they may not go anywhere important—perhaps drift away in the air and not be inhaled or ingested by anyone. But one of these variants might just get inhaled and attached to the correct cell, which it then orders to reproduce trillions upon trillions of itself. And if these are lucky enough to be inhaled by a number of different people, the new variant starts to spread. If it doesn't make people as sick, it can spread stealthily. If it attacks different cells, it can attack different age groups or different parts of the body. If it is more deadly, then it becomes more noticeable.

The following graphic demonstrates the 3,899 genomes that were samples showing mutation variants taken during a thirteen-month period through January 2021.

Showing 3899 of 3899 genomes sampled between Dec 2019 and Jan 2021

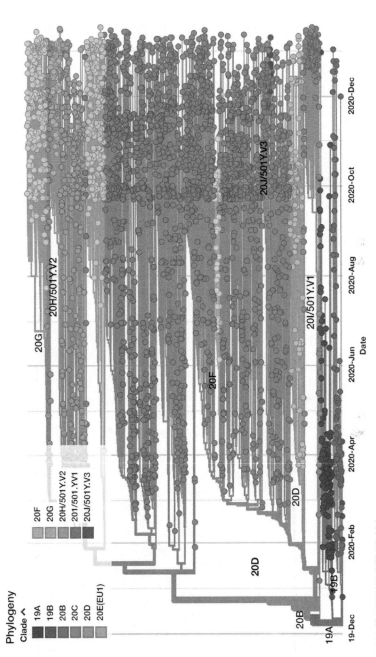

While black and white fails to do this graph justice, it still illustrates the incredible mutation experience the SARS-CoV-2 has. And this is not unexpected of a single-strand RNA. Their very construction allows—actually encourages—mutations. Many of the mutations will be failures, either not lucky enough to penetrate a cell and reproduce or able to penetrate a cell and reproduce but not be passed along through human contact with others; in that case, the mutation line stops right then. But with millions of people infected, the mutations that occur have plenty of opportunity to happen in a person who *is* visiting friends and family—and bingo! The mutation suddenly starts spreading.

There is no doubt that the SARS-CoV-2 strain originated in bats. It probably moved from them through another animal about ten to fifteen years ago, then very recently into humans, possibly from contact with that animal in the "wet market" in Wuhan, China. Probably the disease was noticed in animal farms as the Chinese government suddenly reversed its policy of encouraging wild animal farming and offered to buy back from farmers an initial list of fourteen species of animals. The "offer" (another way of saying "command") was made in Guangdong, Yunnan, and Guangxi Provinces—the most likely source of the contaminated animal that started this mess in the Wuhan wet market. That buy-back offer, not only costing millions of dollars but also destroying a segment of the economy that the Chinese government had been underwriting, is the biggest clue to the government's admission of a disastrous policy it had adopted—encouraging the raising of wild meat for consumption. It is very good evidence of the spread to humans from one of these animals.

Or could this have been an accidental release from the biology laboratory in Wuhan? We may never know.

CHAPTER 7

HOW DANGEROUS IS SARS-COV-2?

Generally, early in one of the classic pandemics of past ages, the dangers from the new disease became readily apparent. Most of them caused an almost immediate horrible, tragic death, and the total numbers and percentage succumbing to the disease were extremely high—much greater than 20 percent. Stuff like that gets your attention real fast.

However, the 1918 pandemic influenza, a disease with ten times the mortality rate of Covid-19, was not all that easy to initially spot nor to understand the terrible significance that it would bring, with over 675,000 in the United States and possibly 50 million worldwide dead in a two-year period.

There are several reasons why admitting the significance of a disease is avoided or ignored.

Such an admission means some action of equal scale must take place, which, of course, comes at a price—sanitation improvements, air flow modifications, disruption of business (work force quarantine, impounded trade goods), and, in the modern era, testing and vaccine development as well as the cost of new antibiotics and treatments.

The advantage in the modern era is we can rapidly identify the causative organism and develop specific treatments and preventions. The disadvantage is the more rapid worldwide spread via air travel. What used to take months to spread across a continent can now spread within hours. We also have reporting systems that should be able to pick up increased disease incidence. However, this can be delayed by a failure to report an observation, such as the muffled early warnings from Wuhan, China, as seen with SARS-CoV-2.

Even in 2021 in the United States there was strong dissenting opinion about the incidence of this disease. One concern was the issue that hospitals are paid a higher rate when a patient is diagnosed with Covid-19. Minnesota State Senator Scott Jensen, a family physician, spoke with Fox News host Laura Ingraham on April 8 about the idea that the number of Covid-19 deaths may be inflated. Senator Jensen stated, "I would remind him [Dr. Fauci] that anytime health care intersects with dollars it gets awkward. Right now Medicare has determined that if you have a Covid-19 admission to the hospital, you'll get paid $13,000. If that Covid-19 patient goes on a ventilator, you get $39,000, three times as much. Nobody can tell me after thirty-five years in the world of medicine that sometimes those kinds of things impact on what we do." This higher rate of pay could account for an overdiagnosis being reported.

I have been on two different hospital executive committees for a total of over thirty years. Coding is one of the most examined aspects of hospital management performed routinely by a number of government agencies. Undercode, and the organization could go broke. Overcode, and I guarantee the organization *will* go broke. Medicare routinely examines hospital billing using a relatively small sample, usually about thirty charts. If they detect an overbilling, they will calculate the percentage of that overbilling in their small sample and then apply it to *all* the hospital Medicare billing for a very extended period of time. The result is catastrophic. If the auditors pick up anything suspicious suggesting purposeful overbilling, significant penalties can even result in criminal charges.

Medicare—the federal health insurance program for Americans 65 and older—does pay hospitals in part using fixed rates at discharge based on a grouping system known as diagnosis-related groups.

The Centers for Medicare & Medicaid Services has classified Covid-19 cases with existing groups for respiratory infections and inflammations. Exact payments vary, depending on a patient's principal diagnosis and severity, as well as treatments and procedures. There are also geographic variations.

An analysis by the Kaiser Family Foundation looked at average Medicare payments for hospital admissions for the existing diagnosis-related groups and noted that the "average Medicare payment for respiratory infections and inflammations with major comorbidities or complications in 2017 . . . was $13,297. For more severe hospitalizations, we use the average Medicare payment for a respiratory system diagnosis with ventilator support for greater than 96 hours, which was $40,218."

It is true, however, that the government will pay more to hospitals for Covid-19 cases in two ways: by paying an additional 20 percent on top of traditional Medicare rates for Covid-19 patients during the public health emergency, and by reimbursing hospitals for treating uninsured patients with the disease (at that enhanced Medicare rate). Both of those provisions stem from the Coronavirus Aid, Relief, and Economic Security Act, or CARES Act.

In summation, the CARES Act created the 20 percent add-on to be paid for Medicare patients with Covid-19. The act further created a $100 billion fund that is being used to financially assist hospitals—a "portion" of which will be "used to reimburse healthcare providers, at Medicare rates, for COVID-related treatment of the uninsured," according to the US Department of Health and Human Services. The question then becomes whether this has caused an increase in diagnosis of Covid-19 in hospitalized patients and the subsequent reporting of a Covid-19 death if they died.

Many estimates have also looked at underreporting. As 40 percent to maybe 80 percent of some age groups who have the illness have no symptoms, these groups—if not tested—are not reported. And while deaths of people with coronary disease can be reported as a death from SARS-CoV-2 if they are infected with it, some deaths in undiagnosed persons are not counted. Estimates seem to usually result in a canceling figure—a 20 percent overreporting and a 20 percent underreporting.

Any suggestion that the disease is imaginary or overreported will eventually fade as the body count increases. And it will increase. This disease is not going away very soon. Not unless we can reach herd immunity, as discussed in chapter 4.

FATALITY RATES

It is well known that there are risk factors that increase a person's chance of dying from Covid-19. What is not as well known are the risk factors for severe illness or complications such as becoming a "never-ender" or a rebound patient. It is still unknown how long immunity will last to prevent reinfection, although the best guess is probably six to twenty-four months of immunity depending on the level of immune response from either the disease or immunization.

In an article in *Nature* magazine, calculations were made by age group and sex, which are displayed on the following table.[1]

COVID Infection-Fatality Rates by Sex and Age Group
(Numbers are shown as percentages)

Age group	Male	Female	Mean
0-4	0.003	0.003	0.003
5-9	0.001	0.001	0.001
10-14	0.001	0.001	0.001
15-19	0.003	0.002	0.003
20-24	0.008	0.005	0.006
25-29	0.017	0.009	0.013
30-34	0.033	0.015	0.024
35-39	0.056	0.025	0.040
40-44	0.106	0.044	0.075
45-49	0.168	0.073	0.121
50-54	0.291	0.123	0.207
55-59	0.448	0.197	0.323
60-64	0.595	0.318	0.456
65-69	1.452	0.698	1.075
70-74	2.307	1.042	1.674
75-79	4.260	2.145	3.203
80+	10.825	5.759	8.292

This table indicates the increasing mortality risk for males over females, starting at age 20 and significantly increasing with age—the risk of death basically doubling every five years with infection over the age of 19. Thus, for every 100,000 males who contract the disease who are 25 years of age, 170 will die. For every 100,000 males over 80 with the disease, approximately 10,825 will die.

Share of deaths　　　　**Share of population**

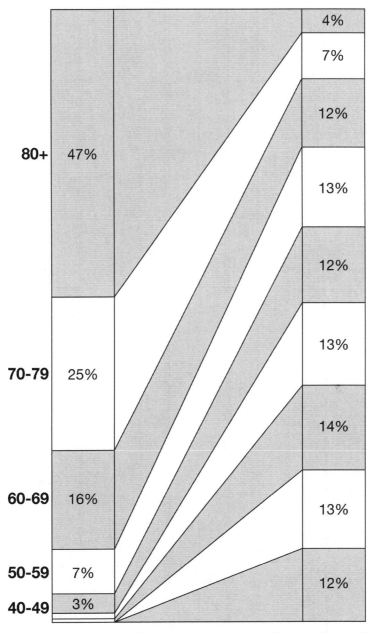

	Share of deaths	Share of population
80+	47%	4%
		7%
		12%
70-79	25%	13%
		12%
		13%
60-69	16%	14%
		13%
50-59	7%	12%
40-49	3%	

This graph illustrates the share of deaths per share of population identified due to Covid-19 as of mid-February 2021.

A *Journal of the American Medical Association* (*JAMA*) article computed how many people were asymptomatic carriers and known infected persons by regions of the United States at the end of April 2020 to establish an accurate case fatality ratio at that time. The authors estimated nontested asymptomatic carriers into their regional estimates based on the regional serology tests. Their conclusion was that for all age groups the case fatality rate was 0.0065.[2]

By mid-January 2021, the case fatality rate in the United States was a fairly steady 0.016, an obviously higher figure.[3] The major contribution of the *JAMA* article, however, was to calculate the number of asymptomatic carriers. The number of asymptomatic, or unknown and unreported carriers, would greatly reduce the actual case fatality rate. That difference is quite high, and, typical of this disease, many data points are simply unknown. Even the fatality rate can be a point of argument and contention. Regardless, as the number of deaths climbs to 1 million, the damage becomes blatant.

Analysis of case fatality ratio (CFR) data comes with a number of challenges. If only the sickest people are tested and therefore diagnosed, CFRs may be artificially high. CFRs also will be skewed in groups who have a higher risk of death, including older people or people with other health problems such as diabetes and hypertension.

An excellent source of up-to-date, country-by-country case fatality rate data may be found at the Our World in Data website.[4]

The percentage of fatalities in the United States reported by ethnicity and race compared with the percentage of the population of these groups has shown alarming disparities.

The disparity between ethnicity/race and proportions dying from Covid-19 has shifted, most likely based on behavior activity. Early in the pandemic with the strict lockdowns, many minorities found themselves at a disadvantage in that they had jobs that prevented lockdown and were bringing the disease back to multigenerational families. As the lockdowns loosened and death totals rose, those enjoying social events like beaches, bars, and parties shifted into white communities, and their percentage of the total deaths normalized against the total population data. In other words, by purposely dropping social distancing, they caught up to those who could not do otherwise.

Share of deaths   **Share of population**

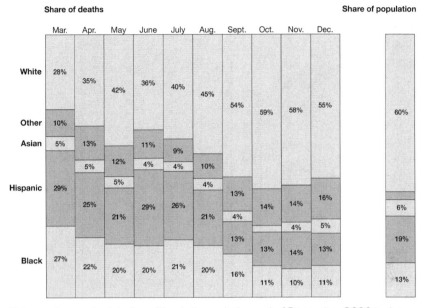

This graph reports data from March through the end of December 2020 in the United States.

A study looking at the association of race and mortality among patients with coronavirus found that there was no significant difference between mortality of Black and white hospitalized patients.[5] The importance of this study was the confirmation that being Black did not put you at higher risk for illness or death from a genetic basis, but apparently it did from a socio-economic basis statistically. The higher percentages of risk for Black, Hispanic, and Asian people was attributed to working conditions (many in essential jobs or labor conditions that did not allow them to shelter), a higher percentage living in multi-family units (placing larger numbers of family and more elderly family at risk when the disease was brought home), and a greater lack of medical care for comorbid conditions. The data is basically driven by unequal infection rates from a social disadvantage, not from a difference in genetics.

The latest data regarding ethnic disparities in SARS-CoV-2 disease statistics for the United States can be found in tabular and graphic form at The COVID Tracking Project.[6] For an extensive breakout of United Kingdom ethnic disparities and risk factors, refer to the article by Claire Niedzwiedz in *BMC Medicine* titled "Ethnic and socioeconomic differences in SARS-CoV-2 infection: prospective cohort study using UK Biobank."[7]

CHAPTER 8

TYPES OF VACCINES

WHOLE VIRUS VACCINES

These are the most traditional types of vaccines. They have been used for a long time, and most of us have had these kinds of vaccines.

They fall into two categories: inactive virus vaccines and live, attenuated virus vaccines.

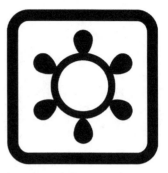

The inactive virus is grown in large quantities in cells, and then killed, often with a chemical such as formaldehyde, or physically killed with heat or radiation. Two of the flu vaccines are made this way, by being grown in either chicken eggs or mammalian cells and then inactivated.

Inactivated virus

Current examples of inactivated vaccines include inactivated poliovirus (IPV) vaccine, whole cell pertussis (whooping cough) vaccine, rabies vaccine, and the hepatitis A virus vaccine.

Unlike live virus vaccines, this type of vaccine can be safely given to people with weakened immune systems.

Unfortunately, they do not provide as strong an immune response as a live virus. Usually, booster shots at regular intervals are required to maintain immunity. As viruses are difficult to grow in large quan-

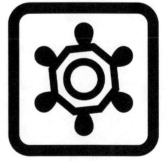

tities, this system does not allow rapidly increasing manufacturing, as with other kinds of vaccines.

Live, attenuated viruses are also grown in cells, but instead of being killed they're genetically "weakened" so they can't infect cells and reproduce as effectively. Traditionally, this was done by getting the virus to grow in and adapt to an environment different from the one they normally infect. That's the approach

Live, attenuated virus

used for vaccines such as varicella (chickenpox) or yellow fever. The SARS-CoV-2 vaccine candidates of this type use a high-tech genetic engineering approach called "codon deoptimization," where the virus is rebuilt from scratch, incorporating targeted mutations that weaken it. The immune response is similar to a real infection, normally providing long-lasting protection after one dose, even lifelong.

These vaccines are not used in people with depressed immune systems from illness or if immunosuppressed after organ transplants. The preparation of these vaccines requires that large quantities be grown in cell cultures, a process that takes a long time. Because these vaccines are live, they require refrigeration, increasing issues with cold-chain storage and distribution.

Examples of live, attenuated vaccines include the measles, mumps, and rubella vaccine (MMR) and varicella (chickenpox) vaccine.

VACCINES THAT TARGET PART OF A VIRUS

Vaccines that are made from parts of the virus, such as specific proteins, can cause an immune response to that specific protein, thus killing a viral threat. In the case of the SARS-CoV-2 virus, the protein chosen to attack is the spike protein in the current vaccines. That is important, as this spike is what the virus uses to attach to the cell it is attacking. Producing an immune response to the spike causes the SARS virus to become harmless.

The differences in the various vaccines causing immunity to the spike protein are the method by which the body is tricked into producing its immune response. Somehow just the spike protein itself must get into the body to cause an immune reaction to it. Some vaccines directly inject a fragment of this protein. Others cause the person receiving the vaccine to manufacture the spike protein internally so their body will then form an immune response against it. These vaccines use a carrier DNA or RNA coded so that the patient will manufacture the spike protein and then form the immune response against it and, of course, against

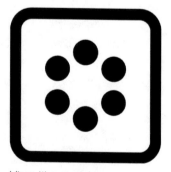

Virus-like particles

the real SARS-CoV-2 virus, if it shows up all covered with its spikes.

Virus-like particles (VLPs) are vaccines in which the protein is made outside the body and then used as a vaccine. With VLPs, the proteins self-assemble into particles that are intended to look like viruses to the human immune system.

Some vaccines on the market that use VLPs include vaccines for HPV (human papilloma virus) and hepatitis B. While this type of vaccine may produce stronger immune responses than regular subunit vaccines, they are hard to produce in large quantities.

VLPs have surface structures resembling the SARS-CoV-2 virus that cause an immune response, killing the virus. They carry no genetic information that can replicate itself and are therefore extremely safe.

Examples of current vaccines that use this technology are two hepatitis B vaccines: GlaxoSmithKline (GSK) Energix™ and Merck Recombivax™. These are among the best-selling and most efficient vaccines being used in the world today. In the United States human papilloma virus infects 24 to 40 million men and women—and HPV has been shown to cause 100 percent of cervical cancers. Merck's virus-like protein vaccine Gardasil™ is approved for use in the United States, and GSK's vaccine Cervarix™ is approved in the European Union and probably soon in the United States.

Virus-like particle vaccines are being developed for such diverse problems as prevention of Norwalk virus gastroenteritis, nicotine dependence, hypertension, and Alzheimer's disease. The safety is remarkable and the potential unlimited.[1]

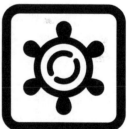

Nonreplicating viral vector

A virus can be engineered to carry pieces of a virus, such as SARS-CoV-2, but not replicate it when it enters a person and cause the carrier disease, resulting in the formation of immunity to the piece of virus they carry. When they are modified to carry a gene from a disease-causing virus, such as the coronavirus spike protein, they can provoke an immune response specifically to that protein.

The nonreplicating viral vectors used by Covid-19 vaccine candidates include adenoviruses, MVA (modified vaccinia Ankara, a weakened pox virus), parainfluenza, and rabies. While that sounds terrifying, it is safe and may generate a more powerful immune response than protein subunit vaccines. They also are stable and do not require extremely low temperature storage.

If someone has already been exposed to the carrier virus, their immune system may reject this vaccine and it would not have a chance to work. These vaccines still require a long process to culture, and making large quantities would be more difficult than other techniques. As each virus can infect only one cell, large quantities of the virus need to be grown and injected (more than a billion copies of viral vectors are used in a single dose of vaccine), adding to production time to manufacture such a concentrated vaccine. These vaccines do not replicate, which significantly reduces the pathogen-specific immune response. Therefore more vaccine doses are required, and it takes longer to get the desired protection. But when protection *is* achieved, it can induce a strong CD8+ T cell–mediated as well as antibody-mediated immune response.

Like nonreplicating viral vectors, replicating viral vectors carry the gene for a protein from the virus you want to protect against, such as the spike protein from SARS-CoV-2, but they are either weakened or don't cause symptoms in humans. They don't actually contain antigens but rather use the body's own cells to produce them. The coding they carry can provide instructions for the human body to make the spike protein, or it may just carry the spike protein

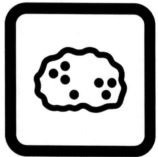

Replicating viral vector

on its surface. The replicating viral vectors used in Covid-19 vaccine candidates include weakened versions of influenza and measles, as well as viruses that cause animal diseases such as horsepox and VSV (vesicular stomatitis virus). They produce new viral particles in the cells they infect, which then go on to infect new cells that will also make the vaccine antigen. There are no replicating viral vector vaccines currently on the market to treat SARS-CoV-2.

The vaccine that has been approved for use against Ebola is the viral vector vaccine rVSV-ZEBOV™ made by Merck.

RNA vaccines carry the genetic instructions (thus messenger) to make a viral protein such as the spike protein. The patient's cells then use the instructions to make the protein inside the body for their immune cells to notice and then respond to with appropriate antibody production.

These vaccines are not manufactured through viral growth, so large quantities can be produced quickly. These messenger RNA particles are very unstable and must be stored at an extremely low temperature. Examples are the current vaccines approved in the United States for SARS-CoV-2 from Pfizer and Moderna.

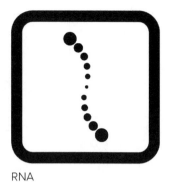

RNA

DNA vaccines are very similar to the RNA vaccines, except that DNA is used instead of RNA. DNA is delivered as a ring called a plasmid. The DNA plasmid platform is safer than conventional vaccine approaches as the plasmids are nonliving and nonreplicating; thus there is no risk for reversion to a disease. Multiple studies have demonstrated the safety of this technique. The plasmids do not alter the DNA of the target cells but simply cause them to produce the protein required to develop the required immune response.

DNA

Current DNA Vaccine Clinical Trials

Phase	No.	Vaccine Targets
I	31	HIV treatment and prevention, influenza, HPV, cancer (metastatic breast, B cell lymphoma, prostate, colorectal), hepatitis B, hepatitis C, malaria
I/II	7	HIV treatment, cancer (prostate, colorectal), hepatitis B, hepatitis C, HPV, malaria
II	5	Cancer (prostate, melanoma), HIV treatment, hepatitis B

Note: HIV, human immunodeficiency virus; HPV, human papillomavirus

There are DNA vaccines currently in phase I, I, and III trials for SARS-CoV-2 vaccines as well.

If successful, these vaccines should have multiple benefits. They are being designed to deal with some diseases that have been refractory to other vaccines, and they would be quick to manufacture at relatively low cost. They also would be stable at room temperature.

In the protein subunit type of vaccine, the protein is made outside the body by breaking whole viruses into nonviable pieces using detergent or a solvent such as ether. This is also being done using another method, called "recombinant" genetic technology, during which the gene for a protein is inserted into another organism to grow the protein in large quantities. These vaccines are sometimes referred to as "acellular vaccines."

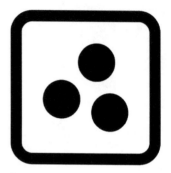

Protein subunit

Because they may not generate as strong an immune response as whole virus vaccines, an additional compound called an adjuvant may need to be included to boost a patient's immune response.

The subunit fragments are incapable of causing disease. They are made to cause specific immune responses. Examples are: protein subunit vaccines containing specific isolated proteins from viral or bacterial pathogens; polysaccharide vaccines containing chains of sugar molecules (polysaccharides) found in the cell walls of some bacteria; or conjugate subunit vaccines, which bind a polysaccharide chain to a carrier protein to try and boost the immune response. Only protein subunit vaccines are being developed against the virus that causes Covid-19.

Many subunit vaccines are already in widespread use, such as the hepatitis B and acellular pertussis vaccines (protein subunit), the pneumococcal polysaccharide vaccine (polysaccharide), and the MenACWY™ vaccine, which contains polysaccharides from the surface of four types of the bacteria that causes meningococcal disease joined to diphtheria or tetanus toxoid (as a conjugate subunit).

VACCINE ADJUVANTS

An adjuvant is a compound added to a vaccine that enhances its ability to trigger an immune response. Various aluminum-containing adjuvants have been in use since the 1930s, as trace amounts of aluminum in vaccines are not readily absorbed by the body. The body's immune system picks up that a foreign body is present and is activated by the presence of the adjuvant, and that response is directed not at the adjuvant but at the foreign protein that has been injected with it. Think of it as sort of a "kick-starter" to activate the whole system. Alum was the only adjuvant known to work for years, but the concept of a kick-starter being added to a vaccine has certainly generated a lot of research.

Vaccines contain very small amounts of other ingredients—some added for a specific purpose—such as preservatives, stabilizers, and antibiotics. Sometime residual materials, such as cell culture material like egg protein, might be found. For a list of adjuvants currently in vaccines, refer to "Adjuvants and Vaccines" at the CDC website.[2]

When a person has a reaction to a vaccine, sometimes that reaction is to one of these ingredients. This is particularly true if the reaction is a local reaction or a generalized severe anaphylactic reaction. If you have a significant allergic reaction to a vaccine, it pays to know what ingredients are in that vaccine. For a full list, refer to "Vaccine Excipient Summary: Excipients Included in U.S. Vaccines, by Vaccine" (February 2020) at the CDC website.[3]

CURRENT SARS-COV-2 VACCINES

By early 2021 the United States had approved three vaccines while other countries had approved vaccines from a number of manufacturers using variations of the "platforms" described above. The messenger RNA (mRNS) vaccines approved initially in the United States, from Pfizer and Moderna, are too complicated to store and use in most of the world, so eventually heat-stable vaccines and those requiring only one injection to initiate immunity will become the predominantly used vaccines. It will take two years to understand the length of time various vaccines will provide immunity to determine appropriate booster timetables and to know how often mutations will require vaccine updates.

This is a rapidly moving target and international in scope. The table below gives a list of the vaccines in testing and production worldwide as of mid-February 2021.[4]

Types of Vaccine Platforms

Platform	Type of Candidate Vaccine	Developer
Nonreplicating Viral Vector	Recombinant adenovirus expressing truncated S protein (rADV-S) [106]	International Vaccine Institute (IVI)
Replicating Viral Vector	Recombinant measles virus spike protein [50]	University Health Network, Canada; Centers for Disease Control and Prevention (CDC)
Replicating Viral Vector	MV-SARS recombinant measles virus vaccine expressing SARS CoV antigen [45]	Institut Pasteur
Protein Subunit	Receptor binding domain (RBD) of the SARS-CoV spike (S) protein [48, 105]	Baylor College of Medicine; Sabin; New York Blood Center (NYBC); University of Texas Medical Branch (UTMB); Walter Reed Army Institute of Research (WRAIR); National Institute of Allergy and Infectious Diseases (NIAID)
Protein Subunit	SARS recombinant spike protein plus delta inulin [49]	Vaxine Pty Ltd, Australia
Virus-like Particle	SARS VLPs S protein and influenza M1 protein [47]	Novavax
Inactivated Virus	rSARSCoV-E* [46]	CNB-CSIC; University of Iowa

Platform	Type of Candidate Vaccine	Developer
DNA	DNA prime–protein S437–459 and M1–20 [51]	Institute of ImmunoBiology, Shanghai Medical College of Fudan University, China
DNA	SARS S DNA prime and HLA-A*0201 restricted peptides boost vaccine [52, 53]	Sun Yat-sen University, China
DNA	3a DNA vaccine [54]	State Key Laboratory of Virology; Graduate University of Chinese Academy of Sciences
DNA	DNA vaccine VRC-SRSDNA015-00-VP; Biojector used [71]	National Institute of Allergy and Infectious Diseases (NIAID)
DNA	DNA S protein + DNA IL2 [72]	State Key Laboratory of Virology, University of Chinese Academy of Sciences
DNA	DNA vaccine pIRES-ISS-S1 [73]	Jilin University; Academy of Military Medical Sciences
DNA	M and N DNA vaccine [74]	National Hospital Organization Kinki-Chuo Chest Medical Center; Osaka Prefectural Institute of Public Health; Jichi Medical School; The University of Hong Kong; National Taiwan University College of Medicine; National Institute of Infectious Diseases; Central Institute for Experimental Animals; Pharmaceutical Frontier Laboratory

Platform	Type of Candidate Vaccine	Developer
Nonreplicating Viral Vector	MVA S alone, or MVA-S prime and Ad5-S boost [107, 108]	The Rockefeller University
Nonreplicating Viral Vector	NC protein admixed with MALP-2 by intranasal route and boosting with MVA–NC by intramuscular route [62]	Helmholtz Centre for Infection Research; Technical University Munich; German Center for Environmental Health
Nonreplicating Viral Vector	Heterologous Adenoviral prime boost AdHu5 s AdC7-nS [63]	University of Manitoba; University of Pennsylvania School of Medicine; Southern Research Institute; Fox Chase Cancer Institute
Nonreplicating Viral Vector	VEEV replicon particles expressing the SARS-CoV S [28]	University of North Carolina at Chapel Hill
Nonreplicating Viral Vector	Recombinant DI expressing S protein [66]	National Institute of Infectious Diseases, Japan
Protein Subunit	Recombinant trunctuated S-N fusion protein [60]	Beijing Institute of Genomics, China
Protein Subunit	Recombinant peptide N223 on liposomes [61]	Saitama Medical University; Josai University; Nippon Oil and Fat Corporation; National Institute of Infectious Diseases, Japan
Protein Subunit	Recombinant TM-truncated S protein [64]	Chinese Center for Disease Control and Prevention; Canadian Science Centre for Human and Animal Health

Platform	Type of Candidate Vaccine	Developer
Protein Subunit	Trimeric Spike protein [65]	HKU-Pasteur Research Centre; University of Hong Kong; National Institutes of Health; Centers for Disease Control and Prevention; CombinatorX
Virus-like Particle	Chimeric VLP (S protein SARS plus E, M, and N proteins of mouse hepatitis virus) [55]	University of Texas Medical Branch (UTMB)
Virus-like Particle	Recombinant trimeric S protein [56]	The Johns Hopkins University School of Medicine
Inactivated Virus	Purified inactivated Vero-cell SARS vaccine [57]	Institute of Microbiology and Epidemiology, National Vaccine and Serum Institute; Beijing Genomics Institute (BGI); Harbin Institute of Veterinary Medicine
Inactivated Virus	Formalin- and UV inactivated virus vaccine [58]	Baxter Vaccines, Austria
Inactivated Virus	ß-propiolactone inactivated virus vaccine [59]	National Institute of Allergy and Infectious Diseases (NIAID); University of Virginia
Live Attenuated Virus	Live attenuated vaccine Nsp16 mutant lacking 2'-OMTase [75]	University of North Carolina
Live Attenuated Virus	Live attenuated SARS-CoV MA-ΔExoN [76]	University of North Carolina

Platform	Type of Candidate Vaccine	Developer
Inactivated Virus	ISCV [81]	Sinovac Biotech Ltd (Beijing Kexing Bio-product), Chinese Centre for Disease Control and Prevention; Chinese Academy of Medical Sciences
Inactivated Viral Vector	RABV-SARS [148]	Thomas Jefferson University
Inactivated Virus	whole virus [132]	Sanofi

CHAPTER 9

NEGATIVE TEST OR IMMUNITY PASSPORTS

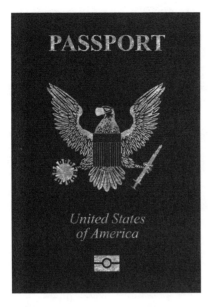

Iceland announced on March 16, 2021, that all travelers who could prove immunization to SARS-CoV-2 (even those arriving from the United States) would not be requested to prove a recent negative test for Covid-19 or be quarantined. Rapidly, most governments adopted similar strategies.
IMAGE COURTESY DAVID R. SCOTT

It has been common, particularly for international travelers, to have to produce a test that "proves" they do not have Covid-19 disease and that is no older than 72 hours prior to departure. Some countries require an additional negative test upon arrival, and even occasionally require a forced quarantine in a particular hotel or designated area (and sometimes simply a quarantine on the honor system).

Eventually this will evolve to having proof of immunization, which will standardize to a format similar to, or become an adaptation of, the World Health Organization Yellow Card.

A proof of immunity would probably have a time expiration, but at this point no one knows just how long immunity from either having the disease, or from any of the various vaccines, will last. Once this is standardized, you can expect that such a card (or electronic app) will be introduced and adopted. While New York was the first state in the United States to produce an immunity app for a smartphone, that will probably become the norm for most countries. It would be easy to calibrate with both immunization and test results to satisfy international entry requirements or for industrial use such as entry to amusement parks, sports events, concerts, transportation hubs, and other venues.

INTERNATIONAL CERTIFICATE OF VACCINATION
AS APPROVED BY
THE WORLD HEALTH ORGANIZATION

CERTIFICAT INTERNATIONAL DE VACCINATION
APPROUVÉ PAR
L'ORGANISATION MONDIALE DE LA SANTÉ

Example of the current (2005) edition of the international vaccination card issued in the United States. This has been primarily used to prove vaccination against yellow fever or meningitis. In the past, it was required by some countries to prove cholera vaccination.

IMAGE COURTESY DAVID R. SCOTT

TRAVELER'S NAME-NOM DU VOYAGEUR

ADDRESS-ADRESSE (Number-Numéro) (Street-Rue)

(City-Ville)

(County-Département)   (State-État)

U.S. DEPARTMENT OF HEALTH AND HUMAN SERVICES

PUBLIC HEALTH SERVICE

PHS-731 (REV.11-91)

COVID-19 Vaccination Record Card

Please keep this record card, which includes medical information about the vaccines you have received.

Por favor, guarde esta tarjeta de registro, que incluye información médica sobre las vacunas que ha recibido.

FORGEY   WILLIAM   W

| Last Name | | First Name | | MI |

GJV 70945 - 51326

Date of birth   Patient number (medical record or IIS record number)

Vaccine	Product Name/Manufacturer Lot Number	Date	Healthcare Professional or Clinic Site
1st Dose COVID-19	Pfizer EJ1685	12/21/20 mm dd yy	Methodist Hospital
2nd Dose COVID-19	EL-3248 Pfizer	1/11/21 mm dd yy	Methodist SL
Other		/ / mm dd yy	
Other		/ / mm dd yy	

The original US COVID-19 Vaccination Record Card

IMAGE COURTESY DAVID R. SCOTT

New York was the first US state to roll out a smartphone app with a QR code indicating an individual's immune and recent testing status.

In the meantime, the aggravation of finding a test that will satisfy the airline or countries on your itinerary—and tolerating a variety of quarantine regulations that will change with the wind—should be expected for the next several years.

The US Department of State has a website that lists all countries in the world with a link to their current specific requirements for travelers with regard to SARS-CoV-2, located at https://travel.state.gov/ content/travel/en/traveladvisories/COVID-19-Country-Specific -Information.html. Checking this site is your best bet to avoid a surprise at your host country. Obviously, check that country's website as well.

All US travelers should be enrolled in the US State Department's STEP program. The Smart Traveler Enrollment Program (STEP) is a free service provided by the US government to US citizens who are traveling to, or living in, a foreign country. Through STEP you record information about your upcoming trip abroad that the State Department can use to assist you in case of an emergency. Enrollment in the program is through the STEP website at https://step.state.gov.

 Smart Traveler Enrollment Program
A SERVICE OF THE BUREAU OF CONSULAR AFFAIRS
U.S. Department of State

CHAPTER 10
SNOW VERSUS BARRINGTON: THE LOCKDOWN DEBATE

MOVING FROM SHUT-DOWNS, "NATURAL IMMUNITY," AND VACCINES TO NORMALIZATION:
The Great Barrington Declaration vs. the John Snow Memorandum

Chapter 12, dealing with pandemics, describes how the implementation of quarantine, social distancing, and health certificates were rigorously enforced during the medieval period. These actions were not readily accepted by the various populations due to the economic hardships that resulted.

In the modern era, immunization has added a powerful weapon to control disease. Indeed, immunizations have eliminated one disease from the planet (smallpox) and almost another (polio). Immunizations can only eliminate a disease from the planet when only humans carry the specific disease and when everyone becomes immune.

Complete lockdowns were prescribed in the medieval period, as they had no other way to slow the spread of epidemic disease. They were not trying to flatten the curve—they were trying to keep the curve from flattening them. Invariably, the curve did flatten them. The "old" pandemics did slow and eventually "die out." But not until the damage they caused was devastating, as can be seen in chapter 12.

At the start of SARS-CoV-2, the only tool in the box was the medieval lockdown and quarantine. In our modern time, the purpose was to flatten the curve; in other words, to slow the spread of the disease so that hospitals would not be overwhelmed and could keep many of the extremely ill alive with respirators, intravenous fluids, and other life-support care. If the medical system were to get overwhelmed, then people would die who might otherwise have been saved.

But shutting down to flatten the curve came with great economic and social cost.

The level of the economic and social cost resulted in the publication of two conflicting opinions on how to manage the situation. First was the Great Barrington Declaration (see Appendix A), named for it having been signed in Great Barrington, Massachusetts. It advocated focused protection. It had become apparent that young people were not even close to experiencing the mortality of the elderly or other identified groups with high morbidity medical conditions. The plan was a proposal to let those with low risk try to assume normal lives without lockdown, therefore limiting the economic and social injury to that group of people. Hence, schools could operate, young people could go out, a certain amount of financial activity could be salvaged in the hospitality and transportation industries, in businesses like gyms, hairstylists, and others providing close-contact services. The elderly would be advised not to participate. The idea is that eventually enough people who have low risk of becoming extremely ill would catch the disease, and that eventually herd immunity would be reached, providing an end to the epidemic.

The potential problem is that while young people do not in general become extremely ill, there are a few who do. And when you are infecting millions of these young people, they do add to the hospitalization rate and the death rate. Further, a small percentage of people with the disease have continued long-term symptoms, which also places a burden on the healthcare system. The major unknown and very worrisome question is, can these asymptomatic young people carry the infection home to vulnerable older household members? And worse, many of the workers at the bars, hotels, etc. might be (and are) members of the high-risk groups. As the young gather, are they dragging the vulnerable into risk?

The John Snow Memorandum was a declaration that obtaining immunity via infection would come at a disastrous cost, and that lockdowns would be essential to prevent an unbearable loss of life (see Appendix B).

Now we have available an option between total lockdown and wide-open disease exposure to obtain immunity, and that is immunization. We also have learned reasonable engineering solutions, such as homemade double or triple face masks or the proper use and value of manufactured masks, airflow technology, shielding, and distancing that can allow increasingly large numbers of persons to safely gather and for businesses to regain function. Combinations of appropriate engineered airflow technology, using specific amounts of online learning at intervals with in-person instruction, and immunization of teachers and students, all can be combined to provide a safe educational experience even in case of a surge of variants and disease activity. Will herd immunity progress via natural infection and immunization to eliminate the need for masks and other social engineering? From studies of past pandemics, the current widespread infiltration of our population by this disease, and the ability of a single-strand RNA virus to mutate, we will probably have a new normal that will include a large degree of appropriate social engineering, which will include masks.

Neither the John Snow Memorandum nor the Great Barrington Declaration are correct if taken as an either/or approach. It will be a combination of acquiring immunization by exposure (unfortunately) and immunization that can save the day. Immunization alone might eventually come to our rescue, while gaining immunity through exposure will prove costly to large numbers of people. But mutating strains, some of which will not be sensitive to available vaccines, means disease will continue. And accidental exposure to large clouds of disease would overcome even those with immunity from either previous disease experience or immunization. Social engineering, such as mask wearing, will be and must be the new norm, but it can be accomplished with minimal financial and social cost.

CHAPTER 11

FOMITES, AEROSOLS, AND FACE MASKS

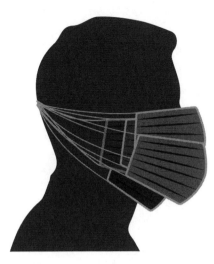

How many face masks should I wear?

What are fomites?

Surface contamination vs airborne?

How far do SARS-CoV-2 aerosols spread?

Can face masks cause harm?

Can face masks prevent disease?

What is the best construction and type of face mask to use?

It's not about how many, but what they're made from and how tightly they fit!

But let's start with fomites. A fomite is an object such as a telephone, doorknob, or article of clothing that may be contaminated with infectious agents (such as bacteria or viruses) and serve in their transmission.

Regarding SARS-CoV-2, the virus particles can independently fall on objects that when touched cause the particles to transfer to another object or to a person's nose or mouth.

The problem is that germs also become encased in mucus, and while these globs do not travel far in air, they certainly fall onto surfaces and provide some longevity to the virus particle's survival.

In the early months of the current pandemic, it was evident that contaminated surface transmission of SARS-CoV-2 was plausible, with the virus being able to remain infectious on surfaces up to days. The maximum time is on stainless steel, plastic, and cardboard. In contrast, on copper surfaces the coronavirus can remain infectious only for approximately 4 hours. SARS-CoV-2 inactivation is possible by using commonly available chemicals and biocides on inanimate surfaces.

The ability of viruses to transfer from a surface to a finger has been studied under low- and high-humidity conditions for room temperature.

Under low relative humidity, transfer of fomite to finger for glass was 19.3% effective. Under high relative humidity, the transfer increased to 67.3%. The transfer also varied greatly with the type of fomite. Under low humidity, acrylic (21.7%) and glass (19.3%) had greater transfer efficiency than other nonporous surfaces like ceramic tile (7.1%), laminate (5.4%), stainless steel (6.9%), and granite (10.2%).

Porous surfaces had very low transfer efficiencies. Cotton (0.03%), polyester (0.3%), and paper currency (0.4%) all had similar low efficiencies of transfer. Under high humidity, the transfer efficiency increased across all materials except for cotton, with little effect on the porous surfaces, but large increases on the nonporous surfaces with acrylic (79.5%), glass (67.3%), ceramic tile (41.2%), laminate (63.5%), stainless steel (37.4%), and granite (30%) all showing marked increases in transfer efficiency. In a more real-world approach, it has been shown that participants performing tasks (such as turning the faucet on/off and holding a phone receiver) that involved inoculated objects showed the highest transfer efficiencies for hard surfaces.

Ethanol at concentrations greater than 70%, povidone iodine, hypochlorite, and quaternary ammonium compounds combined with alcohol are effective against SARS-CoV-2 for surface disinfection. In turn, hydrogen peroxide vapor, chlorine dioxide, ozone, and UV light could be applied to reduce the viral load present in aerosols. These same disinfection practices against SARS-CoV-2 on inanimate surfaces would also be effective

SARS–CoV–2 Surface Decay Calculator

UV Index:	Temperature:	Relative Humidity:
0 ▮ 10	74 ▮ 95	20 ▮ 60
0	87 °F / 30.6°C	22 %

* Note: Temperature (68°F) and relative humidity (20%) input cannot be changed for UV values greater than 0.

COVID Stability:

% Virus Decay	Hours	Days
50% (half-life):	10.01	0.42
99.99%:	132.99	5.54
99.9999%:	199.48	8.31
99.999999%:	265.97	11.08

The Homeland Security's online surface decay calculator for SARS-CoV-2 virus contamination calculates three variables: UV exposure, temperature, and the effect of relative humidity. Access at www.dhs.gov/science-and-technology/sars-calculator.

Although the presence of SARS-CoV-2 on surfaces is possible, even likely, washing hands and regular disinfection practices would greatly reduce the possibilities of transmission of the coronavirus by this potential route of infection. Because influenza does not spread by aerosol but primarily by large droplet and particularly by touching contaminated surfaces and then finger to face contact, surface and hand cleaning is a primary way of stopping its spread. Since SARS-CoV-2 spreads primarily from aerosol, surface cleaning is important, but not as important as preventing the inhaling of super-fine mist particles.

Distance is always a protecting factor from such diverse issues as radiation, heat, and even airborne drift of aerosols. The intensity of radiation and heat decreases at the square of the distance. In other words, the radiation will be one-fourth as strong when you are 2 feet away. Distance also is important with regard to aerosols, as some drop to the floor via gravity, others disperse by air flow, and even direct jets of germs from speaking and coughing are slowed down and eventually stopped by distance. In addition, the virus particles are destroyed by the environment. They are very fragile. Major variables with the airborne survival include the amount of ultraviolet light, the temperature, and the humidity.

A person with Covid-19 can expel 1 billion virus particles per day. While some of these large droplets will fall to the ground and be

SARS–CoV–2 Airborne Decay Calculator

UV Index:	Temperature:	Relative Humidity:
0 ▦ 10	50 ▦ 86	20 ▦ 70
3	70 °F / 21.1°C	36 %

COVID Stability:

% Virus Decay	Minutes	Hours
50% (half-life):	7.29	0.12
90%:	24.23	0.40
99%:	48.46	0.81

The Homeland Security's online airborne decay calculator for SARS-CoV-2 virus contamination calculates three variables: UV exposure, temperature, and the effect of relative humidity. Access at www.dhs.gov/science-and-technology/sars-calculator.

a hazard on a surface, the greatest danger is the aerosolized droplets. These can spread a long way, stay airborne for a long time, and are easily inhaled.

Distance for aerosol spread can be calculated using various laboratory measurements of known mineral powder sizes. It also can be determined for various diseases by observational studies. The mathematical description of the total rate of viable virus particles that would be inhaled by a susceptible individual is provided by the equation below:

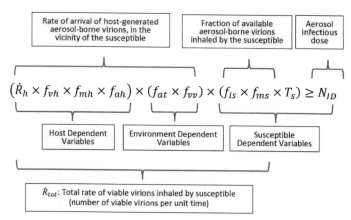

$$\left(\dot{R}_h \times f_{vh} \times f_{mh} \times f_{ah}\right) \times \left(f_{at} \times f_{vv}\right) \times \left(f_{is} \times f_{ms} \times T_s\right) \geq N_{ID}$$

Rate of arrival of host-generated aerosol-borne virions, in the vicinity of the susceptible

Fraction of available aerosol-borne virions inhaled by the susceptible

Aerosol infectious dose

Host Dependent Variables

Environment Dependent Variables

Susceptible Dependent Variables

$\dot{R}_{tot}$: Total rate of viable virions inhaled by susceptible (number of viable virions per unit time)

T_s represents the duration of exposure of a susceptible person to the aerosols from the host, and N_{ID} represents the minimum number of inhaled virions required to initiate an infection in the susceptible.

The contagion airborne transmission (CAT) inequality evaluates the conditions for the airborne transmission of a respiratory infection such as Covid-19. The left-hand side of the inequality represents the total inhaled viral dose, and the right-hand side is the minimum aerosol dose required to initiate an infection in the susceptible. The inequality is satisfied (and the transmission is successful) when the susceptible inhales a viral dose that exceeds the minimum infectious dose. The variables in the model can be segregated in different ways, as shown in the graphic.

A full description of the equation can be found in an article in the journal *Physics of Fluids*, by R. Mitall et al., titled "A mathematical framework for estimating risk of airborne transmission of COVID-19 with application to face mask use and social distancing."[1]

Depending on the size of the particle that the virus particle is embedded in, the airborne distance it will drift varies.

Earlier in the book we discussed the concept of certain concentrations of germs being required to cause illness. The importance of this relates to the use of face masks to decrease the number of germs you breathe to a level that will not cause you harm. While a face mask cannot prevent all germs from entering your body, it can reduce the number that do to below the minimum infectious dose (see chapter 2).

Respiratory Aerosols
Still Air - No Mask

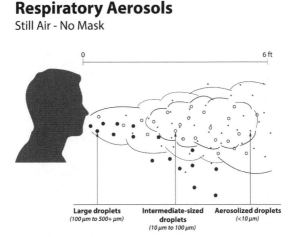

Large droplets	Intermediate-sized droplets	Aerosolized droplets
(100 μm to 500+ μm)	(10 μm to 100 μm)	(<10 μm)

The use of a face mask greatly reduces the distance these particles drift and lessens the force of any breathing jets caused by shouting, singing, etc.

Respiratory Aerosols
Still Air - With Mask

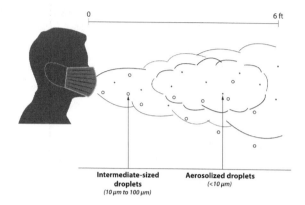

The value of decreased exposure can be illustrated in the following illustration, which indicates risk reduction with exposure between one and two people.

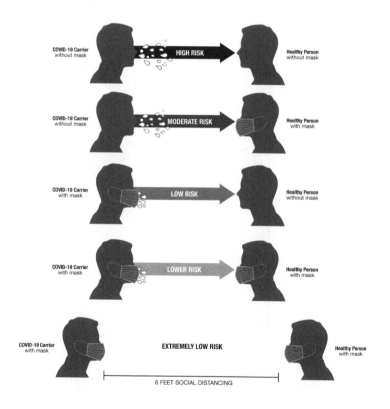

The suggestion that children can safely return to school is based on the fact that children do not develop as high a viral load as adults (due to their having fewer ACE2 receptors in their nasal cavities than adults). Therefore, from both the equation above and epidemiological data (experience in actual practice with schoolchildren), it appears very safe to allow them to congregate with masks at 3 feet in a closed space.

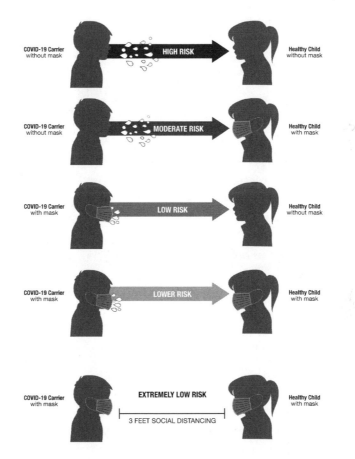

Social distancing and wearing face masks is really all about not swapping air. The University of Minnesota has produced an educational campaign to help spread the "Stop Swapping Air" message (#StopSwappingAir). The concept is to not swap air with people who are not in your pod. A "pod" is a small number of trusted people who are also not seeing others. This term was coined by noted infectious disease expert Dr. Michael Osterholm, and readers are encouraged to listen to his podcast.[2]

Type of fabric, use of filters, numbers of layers, and tightness of fit will obviously influence if and how well masks will work.

Emerging new variants of SARS-CoV-2 will make the proper selection and, if necessary, the continued home manufacturing of masks an especially important topic. Eventually various governments will come out with standards for manufactured masks. They were reluctant to do so during the first years of the pandemic due to lack of adequate supply. Already the Canadian government has suggested a three-layer mask and has provided specific instructions for home manufacture, which are included in this chapter.

The discussion of the use of a mask was initially influenced by not knowing if people could spread SARS-CoV-2 by breathing on each other (they certainly can); then by issues of shortage and the concern that a scared public would all wear masks and dry up the entire supply urgently needed by front-line medical workers; then by wondering if only people with symptoms and thus quite ill could spread it (no one else therefore needing a mask); then by thinking that only heavy particles that fell to the floor would come out of "carriers"; then by realizing that fine aerosol mist could spread it, even from asymptomatic people; and finally by realizing that a lot of people were asymptomatic and that the majority of spread was coming from these people—thus universal masking was the major viable stopgap to be used until immunization or immunity became widespread. Please excuse the long sentence. My excuse in writing it is to provide an excuse for all the confusion about the value of masks.

The problem with mask mandates, and the resulting caseload of Covid-19, is that the mandates do not appear to work. They do not appear to work due to the inefficient actual use of masks and the lag time of a virus that has a high asymptomatic spread before the cases of ill, hospitalized, or dead people show up.

Not only that, but a widely spread disease, especially one that has become more virulent via mutations, is a runaway train. Immunizations and masks provide protection, but not absolutely. We are back to the minimum infectious dose idea. Masked people can tolerate a larger dose in their vicinity but can still become ill—it is just less likely during a specific span of time of masked exposure versus unmasked. The same applies for immunized people. They can withstand a higher virus load in their vicinity than a nonimmunized person, but can still get overwhelmed.

Asymptomatic carriers that spread a disease are a challenge that we fail to understand, as virtually all disease, including influenza, spreads only from symptomatic persons. Faced with a disease that spreads asymptomatically, until you extinguish it from a population, you need to protect yourself from it. This can be partially achieved with social distancing, reducing fomite spread, masks, and immunizations.

Masks are valuable. Some are more useful than others. The international classification of masks was really designed around industrial dust filtration standards.

Mask Type	Standards	Filtration Effectiveness		
Single-Use Face Mask	China: YY/T0969	3.0 Microns: ≥95% 0.1 Microns: ✗		
Surgical Mask	China: YY 0469	3.0 Microns: ≥95% 0.1 Microns: ≥30%		
	USA: ASTM F2100	Level 1	Level 2	Level 3
		3.0 Microns: ≥95% 0.1 Microns: ≥95%	3.0 Microns: ≥98% 0.1 Microns: ≥98%	3.0 Microns: ≥98% 0.1 Microns: ≥98%
	Europe: EN 14683	Type I	Type II	Type III
		3.0 Microns: ≥95% 0.1 Microns: ✗	3.0 Microns: ≥98% 0.1 Microns: ✗	3.0 Microns: ≥98% 0.1 Microns: ✗
Respirator Mask	USA: NIOSH (42 CFR 84) China: GB2626	N95 / KN95	N99 / KN99	N100 / KN100
		0.3 Microns: ≥95%	0.3 Microns: ≥99%	0.3 Microns: ≥99.97%
	Europe: EN 149:2001	FFP1	FFP2	FFP3
		0.3 Microns: ≥80%	0.3 Microns: ≥94%	0.3 Microns: 99%

3.0 Microns: Bacteria Filtration Efficiency standard (BFE).

0.1 Microns: Particle Filtration Efficiency standard (PFE).

0.3 Microns: Used to represent the most-penetrating particle size (MPPS), which is the most difficult size particle to capture.

✗: No requirements.

SOURCE: SMARTAIRFILTERS.COM © 2021 SMART AIR, MODIFIED UNDER CC BY-NC-SA-4.0

As the chart indicates, the filtering ability of all three types of basic masks are relatively identical. For a face mask to work, it must not only filter, but it also must fit well. Because they are loose, single-use face masks are not as effective in preventing virus inhalation as surgical masks that have a stiff nose-conforming stay. And surgical masks are not as efficient as respirator masks, which also can be made to fit more tightly.

Various steps can be taken to give your mask a tighter fit. Having a nose wire greatly improves face mask efficiency. The nose wire is a metal strip along the top edge of the mask. Bend the nose wire over your nose to conform to your face.

Another way of improving a surgical mask (sometimes referred to as a medical procedure mask) is knotting and tying. Knot the ear loops of the mask where they join the edge of the mask, then fold and tuck the unneeded material under the edges. This technique can be seen on YouTube at the following link: www.youtube.com/watch?v=UANi8Cc71A0.

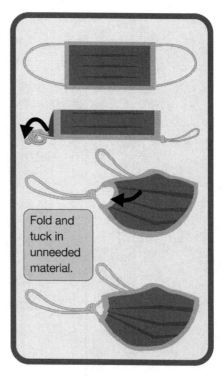

An illustration of the technique described in the YouTube video. The ear loops are knotted, then the crimped material is folded and tucked in.

Fold and tuck in unneeded material.

Masks will always be more expensive than they should be due to this pandemic. Frequently quality masks will be in short supply. A way of solving both quality and cost issues is to make your own.

MAKING YOUR OWN FACE MASKS

Health Canada has made a strong stand stating that homemade masks should be made of at least three layers, including two layers of a tightly woven fabric such as cotton or linen, and a third (middle) layer of a filter-type fabric such as a nonwoven polypropylene fabric, which is washable and works as a disposable filter.

Health Canada makes the clever suggestion that a different cloth be used for each layer, "so you know which side faces your mouth and which side faces out."

Filters and Filter Material

Filters add an extra layer of protection against Covid-19 by trapping smaller infectious particles. When making homemade face coverings, consider using a piece of filter fabric as one of the layers. You can also use a pattern that includes a pocket for a disposable filter.

Disposable filters are widely available for purchase. However, you can also prepare your own filter using nonwoven polypropylene fabric (found as a craft fabric), the nonwoven fabric that's used to make some reusable shopping bags, or a folded paper towel. Do not use plastic film or nonbreathable plastic material as these would interfere with breathing.

These internal disposable filers can be discarded or washed and reused, depending on the material being used. Filters made of nonwoven filter fabrics can be washed multiple times.

Early in the pandemic, my team of nineteen nurses and nineteen medical assistants were quite concerned about making the best possible homemade mask, and we struggled with what should be in that inner filter. We even bought some expensive room HEPA filters, which we destroyed and recut into reasonable-sized insert pads.

For several years I have been packing very contaminated dog bite and bullet wounds with a new bandaging material called Silverlon.[3] Consisting of 99 percent metallic silver bonded to a porous synthetic fabric, its superior wound healing for the deep wounds (decubitus pressure ulcers, diabetic ulcers, and gunshot wounds) that I care for has been superior to xeroform, iodoform, and various other treated dressings. Those treated dressing would not make good middle protective layers due to low airflow capability and the fact that breathing their fumes would be noxious. The company representative offered to send me a few swatches of the material to cut up to use for a middle-piece filter. Then they called to tell me they had decided to manufacture a face mask of their material commercially. While expensive, they are washable, work even better when damp from breath moisture, and cut down on skin acne so commonly encountered when using other masks against your skin. So far my organization has purchased 200 for our use. The downside is that they are expensive—thus back to the topic of making masks at home.

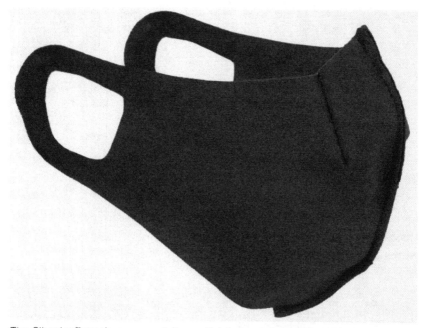

The Silverlon™ mask, commercially available through Argentum Medical, LLC (1-888-551-0188). Silverlon is a nylon material coated with 99 percent pure silver and 1 percent silver oxide. When silver ions are activated with moisture, the ions kill a wide range of pathogens held within the material. The mask tends to sag and requires a tighter outer mask to hold it firmly against the skin, but users experience much less acne when wearing this mask.

HOW TO MAKE FACE MASKS[4]

The Canadian CDC has several methods of making masks, both sewing and nonsewing as described below. Similarly, the US CDC has provided video and written instructions on its website.[5]

Canadian Sew Method*

*© All rights reserved. Nonmedical masks and face coverings: Sew and no-sew instructions. Public Health Agency of Canada. Adapted and reproduced with permission from the Minister of Health, 2020.

MATERIALS

- Two 25.5 cm by 15 cm (10 in. by 6 in.) rectangles of tightly woven cotton fabric
- You can use quilting fabric or cotton sheets.
- Fabric should be thick enough so you can't see light through it.
- One 25.5 cm by 15 cm (10 in. by 6 in.) rectangle of a washable filter fabric
- If a washable filter fabric isn't available, use a third piece of tightly woven cotton fabric.
- Two 15 cm (6 in.) pieces of elastic (or rubber bands, string, cloth strips, hair ties)
- Needle and thread
- Large needle or bobby pin
- Scissors
- Sewing machine (if available)

INSTRUCTIONS

Step 1: Cut out two 25.5 cm by 15 cm (10 in. by 6 in.) rectangles of tightly woven cotton fabric. Cut out one 25.5 cm by 15 cm (10 in. by 6 in.) rectangle of nonwoven polypropylene fabric. Place the rectangle of nonwoven polypropylene fabric between the two rectangles of tightly woven cotton fabric. You'll sew the face covering as if it was a single piece of fabric.

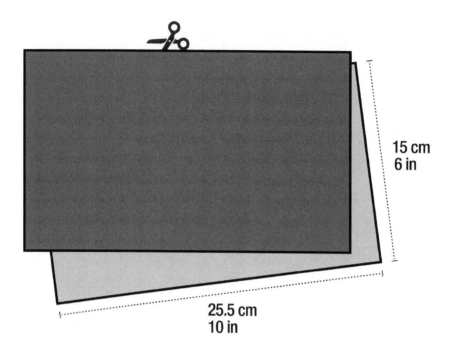

15 cm
6 in

25.5 cm
10 in

Step 2: Fold over the long sides 0.6 cm (¼ in.) and stitch down. Then fold the double layer of fabric over 1.2 cm (½ in.) along the short sides and stitch down.

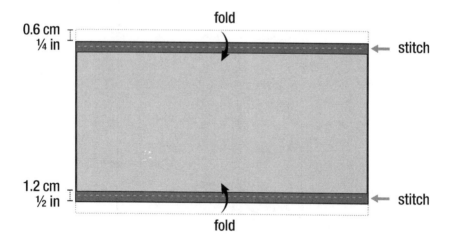

0.6 cm
¼ in

fold

stitch

1.2 cm
½ in

stitch

fold

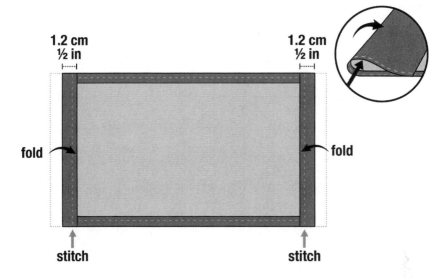

Step 3: Run a 15 cm (6 in.) length of 0.3-cm-wide (⅛-in.) elastic through the wider hem on each side of the face covering. These will be the ear loops. Use a large needle or a bobby pin to thread it through. Tie the ends tight. (Use hair ties or elastic headbands if you don't have elastic. If you only have string, you can make the ties longer and tie the face covering behind your head.)

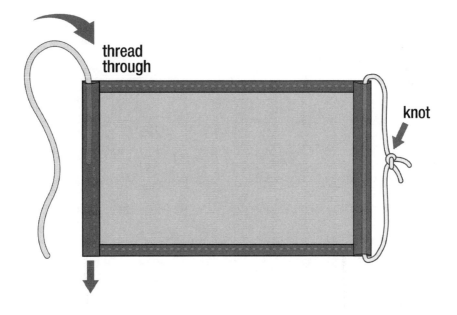

Step 4: Gently pull on the elastic so that the knots are tucked inside the hem. Gather the sides of the face covering on the elastic and adjust so it fits your face. Then securely stitch the elastic in place to keep it from slipping.

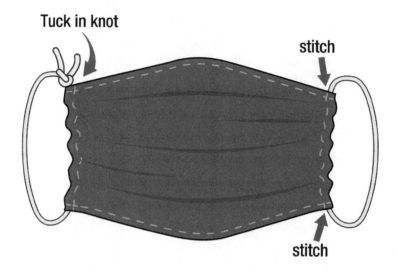

No-Sew Method Using a T-Shirt

MATERIALS
- T-shirt
- Scissors
- Either a piece of nonwoven polypropylene fabric, a disposable filter, or a folded paper towel

INSTRUCTIONS
Step 1: Cut the bottom off a T-shirt (front and back), measuring about 18 to 20 cm (7 in. to 8 in.) from the bottom. The front and back of the T-shirt fabric should be thick enough that you can't see light through it.

Note: For this step and the next steps, you may need to adjust your cut measurements based on the size of the T-shirt you're using.

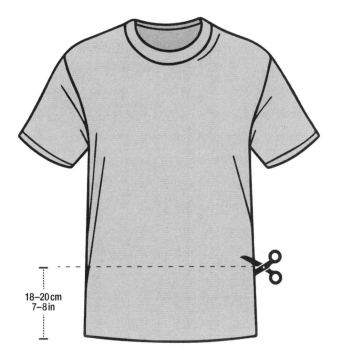

18–20 cm
7–8 in

Step 2: Make two horizontal cuts of 20 cm (8 in.) on the top and bottom of the doubled fabric. Keep at least 1 cm (0.4 in.) width between your cuts and the top and bottom edges of the fabric.

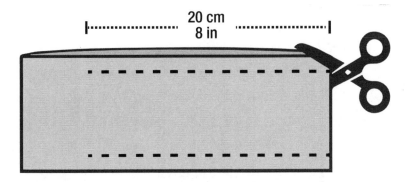

20 cm
8 in

Step 3: Cut out a panel of 5 cm (2 in) from the larger piece of fabric by making a vertical cut between the horizontal cuts. Discard the cut fabric. This will leave you with a C shape.

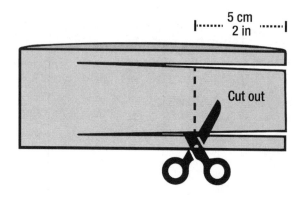

Step 4: Snip the two pieces of fabric at the crease. This will give you a top and bottom set of tie strings. Now you have four strings.

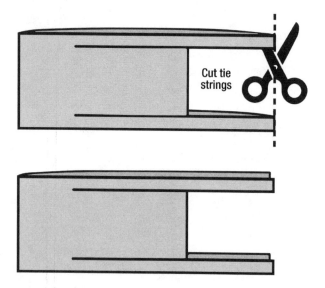

Step 5: Open your fabric so that it lies flat. Place either a disposable filter, a piece of nonwoven polypropylene fabric, or a folded paper towel in the center of the mask.

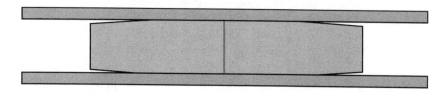

Step 6: Fold the right-hand flap created between the tie strings in half horizontally, toward the center of the mask. The edge of the fabric will overlap the center crease.

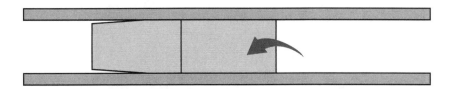

Step 7: Repeat Step 6 on the left-hand side, folding the fabric over the other flap. You now have a mask with three layers of fabric and a filter to cover your nose and mouth.

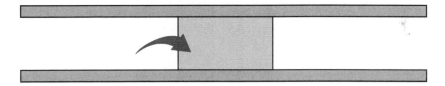

Step 8: Tie one set of strings around your neck, and the other set over the top of your head. The strings that attach over the top of your head will run along your cheeks and above your ears.

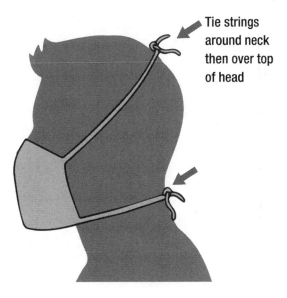

Tie strings around neck then over top of head

No-Sew Method Using a Fabric Square

MATERIALS

- A square cloth approximately 51 cm by 51 cm (20 in. by 20 in.) made of tightly woven cotton
- You can use quilting fabric or cotton sheets.
  - Fabric should be thick enough so that you can't see light through it.
  - Fabric should be a piece of nonwoven polypropylene fabric, a disposable filter, or a folded paper towel
- Rubber bands or hair ties
- Scissors (if you're cutting your own cloth)

INSTRUCTIONS

Step 1: Fold the fabric square in half.

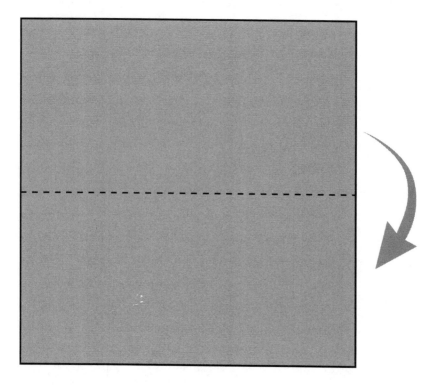

Step 2: Place the filter in the center of the folded square. Fold the top of the fabric down over the filter. Then fold the bottom of the fabric up over the filter.

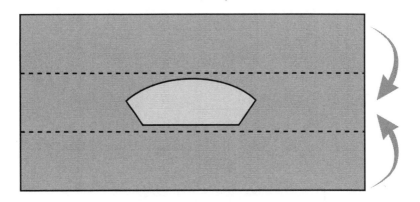

Step 3: Insert the folded cloth into two rubber bands or hair ties, about 15 cm (6 in.) apart.

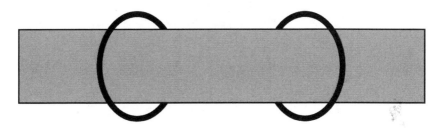

Step 4: Fold the sides to the middle and tuck around the bands or hair ties.

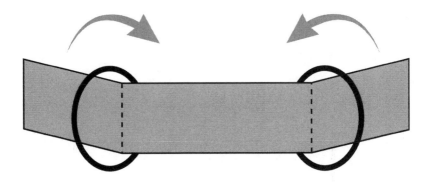

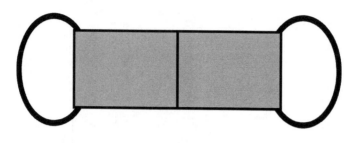

Step 5: Pull the bands or hair ties around your ears.

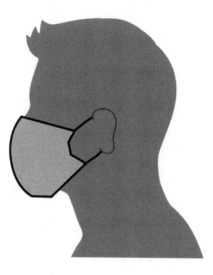

CHAPTER 12

SURVIVING (OR NOT) PANDEMICS

What can we learn from the great pandemics of the past?

What actions did governments take against these massive diseases, and were their actions effective?

Did these pandemics come in waves?

Why worry about pandemics and bioterrorism when we are struggling through a known disaster—SARS-CoV-2 causing Covid-19 disease? Because as bad as it is, it is a piker to what we have seen in the past and what is undoubtedly coming next. The worst of all the plagues experienced by humans have been foisted upon us by Mother Nature.

The millions of people killed by wars have generally had the death toll inflated by diseases and starvation that accompany them. Yes, we can do tremendous damage to each other when we set our minds to it. But for something *really scary*, you need only turn to Mother Nature.

We can learn from our current SARS-CoV-2 experience—and from the past. And if we learn our history well enough, maybe we will not have to repeat it.

Ancient civilizations instinctively developed methods of social engineering—quarantine, restriction of movement—but without effective treatment and immunization, they were left with only natural immunity to bring them through the diseases. The results were inevitable, and they were always disastrous. The disease would hit in waves, with the less vulnerable surviving and attempting to carry on with life as well as they could. But second waves would reoccur until finally everyone had caught the disease and become immune naturally. The death tolls—frequently over periods of decades—were enormous, often leading to the destruction of entire civilizations.

Natural immunity works. But those who survive it bring the disease to others who do not. It is the only choice for a primitive civilization.

Immunizations will always have risk. But the risk of immunizations and the harms that will be experienced by a few pale in comparison to the harm that the unavailability of immunizations has always caused.

There is ample evidence that in prehistory entire civilizations disappeared with only archaeological evidence of their existence. Causes are frequently attributed to climate changes leading to crop failure and starvation, sudden destruction by an unknown enemy, or societal collapse. A local infection causing an epidemic is also a possibility but is difficult to prove. Sometimes a lucky and rare DNA sampling of prehistoric remains might suddenly come to light, and we discover it was an epidemic that caused the collapse. It is certainly a technique that is looking for, and finding, evidence of catastrophic disease at specific ancient Egyptian and Chinese, European Medieval, and New World post-Columbian sites.

The increase in trade routes facilitated disease spread, some of which must have been catastrophic in isolated cities beyond mountain and ocean barriers, and affected vast swaths of humanity. Even in ancient days, the spread of these epidemics happened at a furious pace and the devastation was widespread. During the last 12,000 years, cholera, bubonic plague, smallpox, and influenza have killed between 300 and 500 million people.[1]

These early pandemics show similar patterns of a vicious attack on a disease-naïve population always followed by a series of returning waves. These waves are called "epidemic waves" and are usually a terrible initial onset spike followed by periods of resurgence. (We are all familiar with the term "flatten the curve," which is referring to an epidemic wave.) In every epidemic one must know that the first wave is never the only wave and the second wave can be far more severe than the first. The reason a second and following waves can sometimes be more severe is that the first wave never actually subsided completely. It may have decreased, but the baseline of the disease was still high, and the subsequent waves were surges built on the first wave. This is how SARS-CoV-2 is behaving.

We can learn a lot about the onset of an epidemic, how it was managed, and how our response to SARS-CoV-2 has eerie similarities to these historic events.

Below is a discussion of some of the great epidemics of history—and what we can learn and should take as a warning about each of them. Let's start with the Plague of Athens. Other biblical plagues and ancient Chinese plagues have been reported prior, but historical data for this one allows a much better study of the epidemic features of plagues, with lessons that we had better learn regarding our response to SARS-CoV-2.

PLAGUE OF ATHENS, 430 BC

A lot of historical information is recorded about this early event. This severe illness caused a rapid onset of fever, headache, eye inflammation, fetid breath with sore throat and tongue, and a high mortality rate. It is estimated that 70,000 to 100,000 people died from this disease, which some authorities claim caused Athens to lose its ongoing war with Sparta, a war that was also raging at that time. The Athenians were packed into the walls of their city, thus leading to the proper conditions for a disease to strike. The illness was so terrible that the Spartans withdrew their siege to avoid catching it themselves. Because this war dragged on for years, going through many phases, perhaps this plague wasn't the only reason for the Athenian loss and decline—but it was a nightmare infection that hit hard and fast. It spread beyond Athens, so the Spartans had good reason to scurry away (another reason, of course, was that wars in which Sparta was involved usually had campaign seasons of three months due to the need to oversee their slaves, particularly during harvest).

Plague of Athens Symptoms

- Fever
- Redness and inflammation in the eyes
- Sore throats leading to bleeding and bad breath
- Sneezing
- Loss of voice
- Coughing
- Vomiting
- Pustules and ulcers on the body
- Extreme thirst
- Insomnia
- Diarrhea

Experts have proposed various diseases (over thirty) as the culprit. Typical of diseases entering a community, it returned in 429 BC and then in 427–426 BC.

Most likely causes guessed by historians were typhus, typhoid, or a viral hemorrhagic fever such as the Ebola or Marburg virus. Each of these diseases were possibly endemic to their trade routes, and while all can cause high mortality rates, various descriptions of the victims favor one or the other.

ANTONINE PLAGUE, AD 165

Believed to have been brought into Rome by soldiers returning from war in Partha, the most likely cause of this plague was smallpox. Waves of illness continued for a generation (the classic epidemic curve pattern), eventually peaking in AD 189 when it was recorded that over 2,000 people died daily in the city of Rome. Approximately 7.5 million people died.

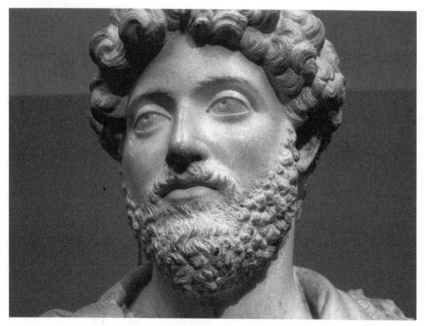

Marcus Aurelius, Emperor of Rome from AD 161 to 180. His decisive political actions during the Antonine Plague saved the empire from collapse even though it suffered 7.5 million deaths out of a population of 40 million.

This caused massive disruption to Roman society. It is lucky for them that Marcus Aurelius was emperor, as he took drastic measures to recruit outsiders into the army and neighboring tribes into vacant farm lands, and elevated the sons of freed slaves into positions of local government—in other words, he took whatever actions were needed and available to him to prevent the collapse of the empire.

PLAGUE OF CYPRIAN, AD 250–271

Striking some eighty-five years later in Ethiopia on Easter AD 250, this plague spread to Rome the following year then to Greece and eventually Syria. It raged over a twenty-year period, killing up to 5,000 people a day in Rome. The death totals for the empire are difficult to estimate, and Rome at that time did not have the leadership of a Marcus Aurelius. The disintegration of military, agricultural, and social structures at that time was probably a major cause of the Roman Empire losing its ability to maintain its frontiers and starting its decline.

St. Cyprian's essay titled *De mortalitate* provides us with our best account of the symptoms and ravaging effects of the pandemic.

Plague of Cyprian Symptoms

This trial that now the bowels, relaxed into a constant flux, discharge the bodily strength: that a fire originated in the marrow ferments into wounds of the fauces: that the intestines are shaken with a continual vomiting; that the eyes are on fire with the injected blood: that in some cases the feet or some parts of the limbs are taken off by the contagion of diseased putrefaction: that from the weakness arising by the maiming and the loss of the body, either the gait is enfeebled, or the hearing is obstructed, or the sight darkened—is profitable of a proof of faith.

Suggested causes were smallpox, typhoid, and Ebola. Sufferers had bouts of diarrhea, continuous vomiting, fever, deafness, blindness, paralysis of their legs, swollen throats, and conjunctival (eye) bleeding. As the description from St. Cyprian, the bishop of Carthage, does not mention pox-like lesions, it is most likely that typhoid fever or Ebola led to these outbreaks.

PLAGUE OF JUSTINIAN, AD 541–549

Contemporary historians claimed that, at its height, up to 10,000 people perished daily, eventually a fifth of the imperial capital Constantinople (present-day Istanbul) from bubonic plague (*Yersinia pestis*). This plague hit in waves that lasted until the eighth century. The death toll over this two-century period has been estimated between 25 and 100 million people, almost one-half of Europe's population at the time.

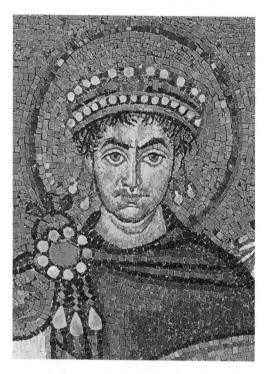

While one of the great rulers of Byzantium, Justinian responded to this plague with very poor management techniques. Not knowing the cause was of course a disadvantage, but not responding to the economic collapse of farm production by loss of labor—or shall we say responding by increasing taxes to make up for the loss of revenue—was catastrophic with regard to assisting the peasant base of the country.

PETAR MILOŠEVIĆ, CC BY-SA 4.0, HTTPS://CREATIVECOMMONS.ORG/LICENSES/BY-SA/4.0>, VIA WIKIMEDIA COMMONS

The genetics of the Justinian plague strain have been localized to central Asia. A skeleton from the Tian Shan mountain range dating to AD 180 of "an early Hun" was identical to the skeletons of German victims from the later period of the disease. After killing up to a quarter of the citizens of the eastern Mediterranean region, subsequent milder waves continued to resurge throughout the sixth, seventh, and eighth centuries, becoming less virulent and more localized. This is a classic pattern for any "new" infectious disease striking a population—an initial crescendo of significant illness and death, then resurgence over a period of years until a significant population immunity dampens it down. This virulent, deadly disease took centuries of waves before herd immunity developed; in some areas it stopped spreading because the population simply ceased to exist. We now have a treatment for this disease, even a vaccine, which we no longer bother using, as we can prevent the spread of rats and their fleas carrying the disease and understand the use of universal precautions when caring for the ill. Remember, this disease has the potential to be dispersed as a bioterrorism weapon, as indicated in chapter 13.

LEPROSY, AD 1100

This disease, caused by *Mycobacterium leprae*, is rare in the United States (200 cases per year), but more common in poor populations in India and elsewhere. The World Health Organization provides free treatment, which has reduced cases from 5.4 million in the 1980s to 216,000 in 2016. Skeletal evidence dating from 2,000 BC in India and Pakistan shows evidence of this disease. It was described by Hippocrates in 460 BC. In the Middle Ages in Europe the disease spread horrifically, resulting in numerous sanitariums and in many countries leper colonies (even including in Hawaii in the 1800s) being built.

There are four strains of this disease, which have allowed epidemiologists to construct a reasonable idea of how this disease spread in ancient and modern days. It can be spread person to person by aerosol, but not very aggressively. The R naught for this disease is very low. But cramped slum conditions can foster the spread even of a disease with a low R naught, and indeed this is what happened multiple times, climaxing in incredible numbers. The DNA extracted from medieval remains shows the strains have not changed or evolved since then. A major reason for the decrease in the disease incidence is in part related to better hygiene and the all-important probability of increased population resistance.

THE BLACK DEATH (BUBONIC PLAGUE), AD 1346–1353

Also caused by *Yersinia pestis*, this was a different strain than the one that caused the Plague of Justinian, and it appears to be an extinct strain today. And just as well, as it wiped out over half of Europe's population once again. The disease started in China in the early 1330s and entered Europe through the Sicilian port of Messina in October 1347. Twelve Italian merchant ships returned from a trip via the Black Sea, a key link in the trade route with China. When the ships docked in Sicily, most of those on board were already dead and those few still alive were gravely ill, covered in black boils that oozed blood and pus.

A writer at the time remarked that the citizens drove the Italians from their city, but it was too late. The disease had started ravaging the countryside and "fathers abandoned their sick sons. Lawyers refused to come and make out wills for the dying. Friars and nuns were left to care for the sick, and monasteries and convents were soon deserted, as they were stricken, too. Bodies were left in empty houses, and there was no one to give them a Christian burial."

By August 1348, the plague had spread as far north as England, where it was first called "The Black Death" because of the black, oozing boils.

It disappeared in the winter because fleas, which carry it from person to person, are dormant then. Each spring the plague attacked again, killing new victims. After five years 25 million people were dead,

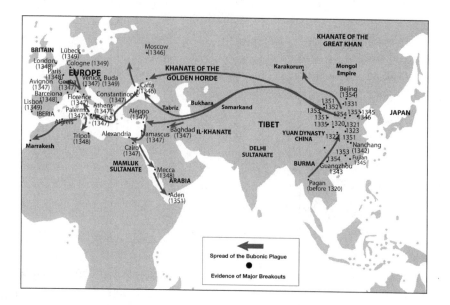

which amounted to one-third of Europe's population. Entire towns were emptied, peasant revolts spread across Europe, and England and France called off their war for lack of soldiers. The human destruction was so terrible it led to the collapse of the feudal system—basically civilization as people knew it.

This disease continued to flare repeatedly for the next 300 years, finally disappearing in the 1600s. Again, as with any newly appearing disease, after causing initial havoc, there were secondary waves of serious impact for years—something we must remember with SARS-CoV-2.

ENGLISH SWEATING SICKNESS, AD 1485–1551

This was a contagious disease that struck England and, later, continental Europe in a series of epidemics beginning in 1485 and lasting until 1551. Death often occurred within hours. Sweating sickness epidemics were unique compared to other disease outbreaks of the time. While other epidemics typically started in cities and were long lasting, cases of sweating sickness spiked and receded very quickly, heavily affecting rural populations.

The disease was described by English physician John Caus, practicing in Shrewsbury, England, in 1551.

English Sweating Disease Symptoms

- Sudden onset with apprehension
- Cold violent shivers for hours, then sweating stage with thirst, rapid pulse
- Giddiness
- Headache
- Severe pain in neck, shoulders, and limbs
- Palpitations, pain in chest/heart
- Irresistible urge to sleep
- Illness lasted for 24 hours, then recovery or death
- Transmission unknown
- Did not attack infants or little children or usually the elderly

It reoccurred in 1507, with a third and more extensive wave in 1517, which ravaged Europe, then in 1528 again starting in Calais, then a fourth outbreak in 1528–1529, then finally again only in mainland England in 1551. When it appeared in a town, it would kill hundreds over a couple of weeks, then fade away.

Historians have debated the cause of the illness, with various authorities proposing it was relapsing fever, but this illness did not demonstrate a skin rash or black scab from a bite site. One of the suggested etiologies was hantavirus pulmonary syndrome, which can closely match the symptoms described. This disease appeared to spread human-to-human, something the hantavirus does not usually do, with the exception of one strain identified in Argentina during both 2005 and 2019.

COCOLIZTLI EPIDEMIC, AD 1545–1548

After an extreme drought, periodic explosions of a disease thought to be a viral hemorrhagic fever killed 15 million inhabitants of Mexico and Central America. Twelve episodes have been identified as being cocoliztli. The largest outbreaks were those occurring in 1520, 1545, 1576, 1736, and 1813. The outbreaks seemed to occur about two years after a rainy period that periodically interrupted a long drought in the area.

The symptoms were depicted by many contemporary writers. One physician, Francisco Hernández de Toledo, who witnessed the outbreak in 1576, described high fever, severe headache, vertigo, black tongue, dark urine, dysentery, severe abdominal and chest pain, head and neck nodules, neurologic disorders, jaundice, spotted skin, and profuse bleeding from the nose, eyes, and mouth with death frequently within 3 to 4 days of onset.

The death toll was enormous, with this periodically appearing illness claiming from 5 to 15 million people. Initially it appeared to primarily affect the Indian population, sparing the Spanish colonialists. Subsequent waves starting twenty-five years later did not spare the Spanish either. Perhaps the original Spanish conquistadores had an immunity from the Old World, which their descendants obviously

Population Collapse in Mexico

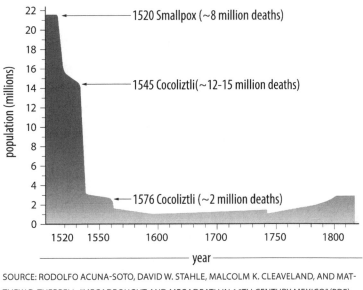

SOURCE: RODOLFO ACUNA-SOTO, DAVID W. STAHLE, MALCOLM K. CLEAVELAND, AND MAT-
THEW D. THERRELL, "MEGADROUGHT AND MEGADEATH IN 16TH CENTURY MEXICO" (PDF),
EMERGING INFECTIOUS DISEASES 8(4): 360–62. ATLANTA, GA: CENTERS FOR DISEASE CON-
TROL AND PREVENTION.

would not have, or perhaps their descendants lived in a deficient social
environment the same as the Indian population—subject to the same
levels of poverty and sanitation.

The cause of this disease is a subject of debate. Diseases that
have been proposed include yellow fever, plague, leptospirosis, hepatitis, malaria, and dengue fever. DNA extracted from the teeth of
ten bodies buried at Teposcolula-Yucundaa in Oaxaca, Mexico, from
a known mass grave, conclusively linked to victims of the Cocoliztli outbreak of 1545–1548, demonstrated *Salmonella enterica* subsp.
enterica serovar Paratyphi C, one of three strains that cause para-
typhoid fever. Yet the symptoms from the historical record are not
a good match. From both a symptom and an apparent relationship
to weather patterns, great interest has been put on diseases that tend
to occur during a two-year rainy season that is otherwise in a megadrought—the weather pattern that coincided with the Cocoliztli epidemics—which would include hantavirus.

A recent experience in North America with hantavirus was an outbreak of a deadly disease among some members of the Navajo Nation in the Four Corners region of the United States, the geographic intersection of Utah, Colorado, New Mexico, and Arizona, in 1993. It infected twenty-six and killed thirteen. It was rapidly identified by a physician as a probable pulmonary variety of hantavirus, based on his experience with this illness, which had infected US soldiers in the Korean War in the mid-1950s. This strain did not spread human-to-human but was most likely from inhaled dust particles. A recent rainy year had caused a mouse explosion in the region, which had acted as the reservoir for the disease.

This disease (Orthohantavirus family) causes two variations of illness: hemorrhagic fever with renal syndrome and hantavirus pulmonary syndrome, caused by Old World and New World hantaviruses, respectively. The renal syndrome is usually more fatal. It starts with high fever, chills, headache, backache, abdominal pains, nausea, and vomiting. Eventually there is bleeding under the skin, low blood pressure, and internal bleeding throughout the body.

The important points that the Cocoliztli experience demonstrated are the incredible mortality rate, the strong evidence of human-to-human spread by aerosol, the speed by which it spread in a civilization where commerce was on foot or by horse, and the fact that this unknown disease recurred multiple times with great ferocity periodically over sixty years (being dormant between killing sprees). It is probably lurking endemically in the Mexican highlands and elsewhere in the world. Were this virus to again mutate, the modern connections of transportation could within days cause a catastrophic spread of a disease that is much more highly contagious than SARS-CoV-2, and by far more lethal. Each time this disease flared in central Mexico, it cut the population in half.

AMERICAN PLAGUES, 1600S

This is the term given for a whole series of disastrous infectious diseases, possibly intertwined with adverse climate change events, that caused the deaths of perhaps 95 percent of the indigenous population of South, Central, and North America.

Unlike the Cocoliztli epidemic described above, the incredible devastation on numerous cultures in the New World was due to a multitude of diseases brought from Europe and then eventually from Africa via slave importation. The devastation that resulted was due to the lack of any immunity in a population naïve to these diseases. Wave after wave swept through, with many of the episodes witnessed and identified by Europeans. Some accurate and good estimates of regional and specific tribal losses have been recorded, but many were unwitnessed, with only the existence of empty lands showing archaeological evidence of once thriving cultures as witness to the destruction.

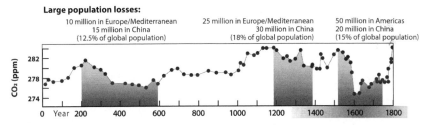

Population decreases and CO_2 decreases recorded in ice cores from the Law Dome over the last 2,000 years correlating with mass human extinction events (Ruddiman, *Earth Transformed,* W.H. Freeman, 2013).

Without modern science and technology, the only means of controlling pandemics were quarantine and social distancing. Additionally, Europeans had built up herd immunity—though the cost had been heavy, actually catastrophic. Unfortunately, the natives were unaware of the notion of quarantine, which Europeans had been practicing since the Black Death three centuries earlier.

There is one certainty about the Great American Pandemic of the sixteenth century. The death toll was frightening. In Texas and Arkansas, the Caddo population numbered 200,000 at the time. The population fell from 200,000 to 8,500 in a century. In 1517 the population of the Timucua in Florida was estimated to be 722,000. In 1596 this group had declined to 72,900. The indigenous populations of South, Central, and North America suffered a decline of 95 percent of their numbers during the sixteenth century.

Diseases ravaging North America included smallpox, influenza, mumps, cholera, and measles. Even bubonic plague swept through Florida and the Southwest in 1545. This series of pandemics depopulated North America in the sixteenth and seventeenth centuries. The virgin wilderness the French fur traders, British colonists, and American settlers found in the seventeenth and eighteenth centuries was a post-apocalyptic wasteland.

Smallpox, or variola, was the most destructive disease in human history because it kept coming back, returning every few decades for generations, devastating Native American societies just as they recovered from earlier pandemics.

Only tiny bands of survivors remained in some areas. The Pilgrims found empty villages and cleared fields ready for plowing when they arrived in Massachusetts in 1620. The European diseases had preceded them by one hundred years.

GREAT PLAGUE OF LONDON, AD 1665–1666

The bubonic plague returned in April 1665, rapidly spreading during the hot summer months. While plague is initiated from fleas carried by rodents, once human-to-human transmission starts, the devastation mounts rapidly. While Europeans had realized the importance of separating themselves from ill patients by either quarantining or isolating the ill, the main method was simply fleeing from cities or other hot spots where the disease was present. This, of course, resulted in significant disease spread.

Over 15 percent of the population of London died that summer, a staggering 100,000 people. What seems like a comic skit by Monty Python of carts rolling through the streets of London calling out "Bring out your dead" was the reality of the Great Plague of London. The following year, in September 1666, the Great Fire of London broke out. It burned for 4 days and consumed a large portion of the city.

GREAT PLAGUE OF MARSEILLE, AD 1720–1723

As mentioned, Europeans had developed a tool—practically their only tool—in fighting the great contagions of the time, and that was the use of quarantine.

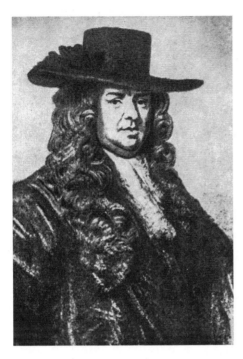

Samuel Pepys's diary from 1660 to 1669 gave us a clear picture of the horrors of the Great *Plague* in London and the governmental reactions. In many respects, the edicts by officials mirrored our current response to SARS-CoV-2, with travel restrictions, quarantines, and social distancing rules—the only difference being the lack of a vaccine. Many of these rules are like those in use in Europe since the Black Death starting in 1346.

The Great Plague of Marseille in 1720 was not an entirely new (or novel) disease thrust upon them. This fierce disease, whenever it appeared, caused the deaths of a significant percentage of everyone in the countryside and was a feared catastrophe. Going back to AD 1346–1353, the Black Death, caused by the same strain of the bacterium *Yersinia pestis*, had been active intermittently in Europe (usually causing devastation a decade at a time) for centuries.

Nobody had mastered the art of the use of quarantine better than the city of Marseille. This technique had been developed some 370 years before during the Black Death. Quarantine, the holding of new arrivals or ill people in a separate holding area for 40 days, was first implemented at the port city of Dubrovnik on Croatia's Dalmatian Coast in 1377.

The people of Marseille had adopted all the precautions. Among the techniques developed in 1377 were:

- A Sanitation Board that established health regulations and monitored evidence of disease outbreak. Documents show that it had been making active recommendations since at least 1622. The first hospital was built and staffed with doctors and nurses. Local doctors were accredited by the Board.

- The Board established a sophisticated three-tier quarantine system. Members of the board actually inspected all incoming ships. These ships were then given one of three "bills of health" depending on the risk of the sailors and cargo. The bill of health then determined the level of access to the city by the ship and its cargo.

- The delegation would board each ship and check its log to determine if it had been at any of the Board's master list of cities throughout the Mediterranean that were suspected of having plague.

- The delegation inspected the crew, passengers, and all cargo. If they found any evidence of disease, or contact with a diseased port, the vessel was not allowed to land at a Marseille dock. There were two tiers of quarantine that were fully functioning.

The first test was demonstrating no sign of disease. If the ship's itinerary included a city with documented plague activity, the ship was sent to the second tier of quarantine at islands outside Marseille harbor. The criteria for the lazarettos (quarantine facilities) were ventilation to drive off what was thought to be the vapors causing the disease, to be near the sea to access the water to clean the ships, and to be isolated yet easily accessible.

A clean bill of health for a ship still required a minimum of 18 days' quarantine at the off-island location. During such time, the crew would be held in one of the lazarettos that were constructed around the city. These lazarettos were also classified according to bills of health. Crewmen from a ship with a clean bill went to the largest quarantine site, equipped with stores and large enough to accommodate many ships and crews at a time.

If crew members were believed subject to a possibility of plague, they were sent to the more isolated quarantine site, which was built on an island off the coast of the Marseille harbor. The crew and passengers were required to wait there for 50 to 60 days to see if they developed any sign of plague.

Only after crews had served their appropriate length of time were they allowed into the city in order to visit the port prior to departure and to have their cargo moved into the city.

So, with this sophisticated system of training, inspection, building of two levels of quarantine isolation for hundreds of sailors, levels of storage, and decontamination techniques for all cargo, what went wrong?

The merchant ship *Grand-Saint-Antoine* arrived in Marseille on May 25, 1720. The vessel had departed from the port of Sidon in Lebanon, after previously visiting Smyrna, Tripoli, and the plague-ridden island of Cyprus. A Turkish passenger was the first to be infected and soon died, followed by several crew members and the ship's surgeon. The ship was refused entry to the port of Livorno, in Tuscany, Italy.

When it arrived at Marseille, it was promptly placed under quarantine in the quarantine station. Powerful city merchants, namely the city's primary municipal magistrate, Jean-Baptiste Estelle, who owned part of the ship and a large part of its cargo, wanted the silk and cotton unloaded from the ship for the great medieval fair at Beaucaire and pressured authorities to lift the quarantine.

The result was an outbreak of plague. Fifty thousand of Marseille's total population of 90,000 died, and an additional 50,000 people in other areas succumbed as the plague spread north.

How was it stopped?

Rigorous social distancing was the only tool that humans had before the discovery of the cause of the disease (in this case a bacterium spread by coughing and close contact), treatment (for which we now have an antibiotic), sanitation (to prevent rats carrying fleas into our presence), immunization (which we now have for those entering a high-risk situation), and, as always when dealing with a serious disease killing many of your neighbors, very vigorous enforcement.

First, they levied the death penalty for any communication between Marseille and the rest of Provence. To aid enforcement they built a stone wall 6 feet, 7 inches high and 28 inches thick across the countryside with guard posts along the inside.

The government built a new, larger lazaretto, ringed the white-washed compound with a double 15-foot-high wall, and required all merchantmen to undergo inspection at an island farther out in the harbor. But of course, the problem had not been with the system but with a person of power breaching the system's well-planned provisions.

General Commissioner Nicholas Roze established a quarantine and set up checkpoints that included gallows to hang looters. He also had five large mass graves dug, and on September 16, 1720, he personally headed a 150-strong group of volunteers and prisoners to remove 1,200 corpses that had been abandoned in the city. Some of the corpses were three weeks old, and contemporary sources describe them as "hardly human in shape and set-in movement by maggots." In half an hour, the corpses were thrown into open pits that were then filled with lime and covered with soil. Out of 150 volunteers and prisoners deployed to fight the plague, only three survived. Roze became ill himself but survived. He organized humanitarian supplies for the quarantined citizens and established another hospital.

In the area touched by this plague, between 25 and 50 percent of the population died. But this death toll, and the length of time during which it raged, was certainly constricted by the aggressive actions taken by the government when compared to the other periods of plague described in this chapter that had happened in Europe and elsewhere before.

No people at any time in history have tolerated quarantine well. Even when the death rate destroyed half the population, these restrictions were met with great resistance. But shy of gallows hanging, many of the techniques of the thirteenth through eighteenth centuries did develop a number of sanitation solutions and social distancing skills that are appropriate to the current day. In fact, virtually all the social distancing (barriers at bars, 6 feet between people, handwashing, quarantine) were outlined in a number of early documents of the period. Perhaps none is better than that published by Quinto Tiberio Angelerio in 1588, included in this book in its entirety as Appendix D.[3] While some of it has very peculiar medieval suggestions, much of it sounds like the CDC playbook.

The disease, plague, or *Yersinia pestis*, has continued to periodically rage across the world. In 1855 it started in China, moved via Hong Kong, then devastated much of Asia including India. In 1960 the Third World Plague Epidemic was considered ended, as only a few cases sporadically occur. In the United States about three to six cases are seen yearly in the western desert. But this disease has the ability, as it has shown repeatedly, to flare, causing large percentages of the population to die. We now have a vaccine and we have antibiotic treatment. With treatment no more than 20 percent of persons catching it should die. And we now know how to quarantine. This is a disease that can be weaponized for bioterrorism use, as discussed in chapter 13.

AMERICAN EPIDEMICS FROM COLONIZATION ONWARD

Along with famine and war, it was disease that decided who survived in the American colonies. Smallpox was the most feared, but malaria took more lives than any other disease. Dysentery was the number two killer of colonists. The next most fatal illnesses were the respiratory complaints: influenza, pneumonia, pleurisy, and colds. After that, the ranking would be smallpox, yellow fever, diphtheria and scarlet fever, measles, whooping cough, mumps, typhus, and typhoid fever.

The fatality rate from disease in colonial times for Native Americans was 55 to 90 percent. An example is the complete decimation of the Pamlico tribe in South Carolina in 1698–1699. John Duffy claims, in his book *Epidemics in Colonial America*, that respiratory diseases weakened and eventually killed more colonists than smallpox.

The major epidemics that hit the North American continent were:

North American Outbreaks and Epidemics, 17th and 18th Centuries

1657	Boston: Measles	1798	Philadelphia: Yellow Fever (one of worst)
1687	Boston: Measles		
1690	New York: Yellow Fever	1803	New York: Yellow Fever
1713	Boston: Measles		
1729	Boston: Measles	1820–1823	Nationwide: "fever" (starts on Schuylkill River, PA, and spreads)
1732–1733	Worldwide: Influenza		

1738	South Carolina: Smallpox
1739–1740	Boston: Measles
1747	Connecticut, New York, Pennsylvania, and South Carolina: Measles
1759	North America (areas inhabited by white people): Measles
1760–1761	North America and West Indies: Influenza
1772	North America: Measles
1775	North America (especially hard in New England): Epidemic (unknown)
1775–1776	Worldwide: Influenza
1778	Valley Forge, PA: Smallpox
1781–1782	Worldwide: Influenza (one of worst flu epidemics)
1788	Philadelphia and New York: Measles
1831–1832	Nationwide: Asiatic Cholera (brought by English emigrants)
1832	New York and other major cities: Cholera
1837	Philadelphia: Typhus
1841	Nationwide: Yellow Fever (especially severe in South)
1847	New Orleans: Yellow Fever
1847–1848	Worldwide: Influenza
1848–1849	North America: Cholera
1850	Nationwide: Yellow Fever
1850-1851	North America: Influenza
1852	Nationwide: Yellow Fever (New Orleans: 8,000 die in summer)
1855	Nationwide (many parts): Yellow Fever
1857–1859	Worldwide: Influenza (one of disease's greatest epidemics)
1860–1861	Pennsylvania: Smallpox
1865–1873	Philadelphia, New York, Boston, New Orleans, Baltimore, Memphis, and Washington DC: a series of recurring epidemics of Smallpox, Cholera, Typhus, Typhoid,

1793	Vermont: Influenza and a "putrid fever"
1793	Virginia: Influenza (kills 500 people in 5 counties in 4 weeks)
1793	Philadelphia: Yellow Fever (one of worst)
1783	Delaware (Dover): "extremely fatal" bilious disorder
1793	Pennsylvania (Harrisburg and Middletown): many unexplained deaths
1794	Philadelphia: Yellow Fever
1796–1797	Philadelphia: Yellow Fever
	Scarlet Fever, and Yellow Fever
1873–1875	North America and Europe: Influenza
1878	New Orleans: Yellow Fever (last great epidemic of disease)
1885	Plymouth, PA: Typhoid
1886	Jacksonville, FL: Yellow Fever
1918	Worldwide: Influenza (high point year)

To augment this list, the current or recent pandemics affecting the world are:

- Asian flu, 1957–1958: killed more than 1 million
- AIDS pandemic, 1981–present day: killed more than 35 million; currently 40 million infected
- H1N1 swine flu, 2009–2010: infected 1.4 billion people and killed between 151,700 to 575,400 per the CDC
- West African Ebola epidemic, 2014–2016: infected 28,616 and killed 11,310

- Zika virus epidemic, 2015–present day
- SARS-CoV-2 pandemic, 2019–present day

The importance of looking at the pandemics of the past is that they all behave the same. There is the initial appearance of the disease, usually a point of geographic entry, and then very rapid spread. Historically these diseases spread quickly over long distances, even with the slow transportation of the Middle Ages through the end of the nineteenth century. The thing that flares them is a crowded city or event, such as an army or a fair. These deadliest diseases of mankind spread from human to human, so that makes perfect sense. They usually initially spread to humans from an animal source, but once in humans then people-to-people interaction takes over.

The pandemics always come in "waves." Some are seasonal, and multiple waves can occur over a short time, even two years, as was the case with the terrible influenza epidemic of 1918.

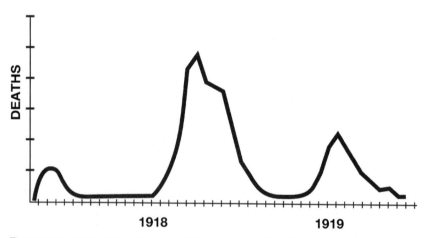

There were three different waves of illness during the influenza pandemic, starting in March 1918 and ending by summer of 1919. It peaked in the United States, with the second wave during the fall of 1918. Most deaths occurred in the second wave.

Other pandemics had waves that lasted a decade at a time and reoccurred over centuries. For example, the Black Death plague had an initial series of waves affecting Europe during 1346 to 1353, but returned in periodic giant waves until the early 1600s.

The cause of epidemic or pandemic waves are argued about and studied, with the cause of the 1918 influenza's three-wave phenomenon still being passionately discussed. The causes of secondary waves are multifactorial. It could be that an initial flare then smolders, spreading among mostly asymptomatic carriers, then erupts secondary to large back-to-school and sports events, large armies forming together, or gatherings of people during summer activities—anything that can bring people together. With a highly contagious disease, even many small family gatherings can cause a snowball effect of asymptomatic spread that then hits a critical mass, finally erupting into plain sight.

Another cause frequently postulated is the germ changing, suddenly mutating to something more virulent, maybe even reinfecting those who already suffered during the first wave. Also, the population might become exposed to a second disease that overlaps the first, creating a second wave of illness and even death that mingles with data from the first. Both are possible scenarios to be added to the asymptomatic spread issue.

Expect mutations certainly with SARS-CoV-2 and waves with these mutations. Refer to chapter 6 concerning mutations of SARS-CoV-2.

CHAPTER 13
BIOTERRORISM

What infectious diseases are at risk of being used in a bioterrorism release?

What is the difference between natural disease epidemics and a bioterrorism release?

Was SARS-CoV-2 a natural disease or an accidental lab release?

There are many natural diseases that can be as deadly as any bioterrorism weapon—in fact, they *are* exactly the same thing as the germ that would be used as a bioterrorism weapon. Some naturally occurring diseases have at times killed half the population of a civilization on their own.

Immense sums are spent by nations to stockpile treatment and preventive vaccines for some of these diseases in case they become weapons. The real danger to humanity is that they are here with us, they lurk in the background, many have suddenly emerged in the past, and they are capable on their own of reemerging to cause havoc again.

The following tables summarize the diseases found in North America and other similar high-risk illnesses encountered throughout the world. Table 1 summarizes the diseases encountered naturally in North America, and Table 2 the diseases of the world.

Bioterrorism is when one of these diseases is brought to you on purpose by some bad actor. Some of these illnesses are rarely seen in North America; others are here but seldom encountered. Some diseases are returning in force due to low immunization rates.

Table 1

Significant Naturally Occurring Diseases of North America with a Potential for Epidemics

Illness	Source/Vector
Anaplasmosis	tick
Babesiosis	tick
Blastomycosis	soil
Coccidioidomycosis	soil
Colorado Tick Fever	tick
Echinococcus	water
Ehrlichiosis	tick
Encephalitis	mosquito
Giardiasis	water
Hantavirus	rodents/soil
Hepatitis A, E	water, food
Hepatitis B, C, D, G	blood, sex
Lyme Disease	tick
Meningococcal Meningitis	people
Plague	rodents/fleas, people
Rabies	mammals
Relapsing Fever	tick
Rocky Mountain Spotted Fever	tick
STARI	tick
Tetanus	soil
Tick Paralysis	tick
Trichinosis	food
Tuberculosis	people
Tularemia	tick, fly
Typhus, endemic	fleas
West Nile Virus	mosquito

Table 2
Significant Infectious Diseases of the World with a Potential for Epidemics

Illness	Source/Vector
Cholera	water
Chikungunya Fever	mosquito
Dengue	mosquito
Malaria	mosquito
Schistosomiasis	snail/water
Tapeworms	food/water
Trypanosomiasis, African	fly
Trypanosomiasis, American	reduviidae insect
Typhoid Fever	water/food
Typhus, Epidemic	lice
Yellow Fever	mosquito
Zika	mosquito

The US government classifies these diseases into three categories regarding their ease of being weaponized:

BIOTERRORISM AGENTS/DISEASES
Category A
1. Can be easily disseminated or transmitted from person to person
2. Result in high mortality rates
3. Might cause public panic and social disruption
4. Require special action for public health preparation

Category B
1. Are moderately easy to disseminate
2. Result in moderate morbidity and mortality
3. Require special enhancements of CDC's diagnostic capacity and enhanced surveillance

Category C

1. Availability
2. Ease of production and dissemination
3. Potential for high morbidity and mortality rates and major health impact

Diseases found naturally in North America that are considered Category A are plague and tularemia, and from Category B typhus fever and various food and waterborne diseases. These diseases have been the cause of worldwide pandemics in the past that have killed millions.

Other Category A diseases (anthrax—the last case in the United States was in 1976), botulism (caused by poor food preservation), and smallpox (now extinct from the world except in certain US and Russian laboratories) are not something you will encounter unless there is a mass bioterrorism release. The viral hemorrhagic fevers are also in this category (Ebola, Marburg, Lassa, and Machupo viruses).

Category B agents encountered naturally are brucellosis, glanders, melioidosis, psittacosis, and Q fever—again diseases that are so rare as to be insignificant unless used purposely as biological agents.

As mentioned above, these are the diseases most likely to be used in germ warfare, either by a major enemy power or by a terrorist group. These can be easily disseminated or transmitted from person to person, result in high mortality rates, might cause public panic and social disruption, and require special action for public health preparation.

Table 3 is a full list of infectious disease by bioterrorism category with availability of vaccine (some experimental but with limited use approval) and treatment.

Table 3

Category A Agents	Vaccine	Treatment
Anthrax (*Bacillus anthracis*)	Available, not commonly used	Ciprofloxacin, levofloxacin, and doxycycline
Botulism (*Clostridium botulinum toxin*)		antitoxin
Plague (*Yersinia pestis*)	Available, not commonly used	Ciprofloxacin, levofloxacin, and doxycycline
	Post-exposure doxycycline	Streptomycin, gentamycin
Smallpox (*variola major*)	Vaccine available in military reserve	
Tularemia (*Francisella tularensis*)		Streptomycin, gentamicin, doxycycline, and ciprofloxacin
Ebola	Vaccine	Supportive care
Marburg	Vaccine in development	Supportive care
Lassa		Ribavirin
Machupo		Supportive care

Category B Agents	Vaccine	Treatment
Brucellosis (*Brucella* species)		Doxycycline and rifampin
Epsilon toxin of *Clostridium perfringen*		Supportive care
Food safety threats (*Salmonella* species, *Escherichia coli* O157:H7, *Shigella*)		Ciprofloxacin, or azithromycin, frequently only hydration and supportive care

Category B Agents	Vaccine	Treatment
Glanders (*Burkholderia mallei*)		Sulfadiazine and multiple others
Melioidosis (*Burkholderia pseudomallei*)		Intravenous therapy consists of Ceftazidime administered every 6 to 8 hours OR Meropenem administered every 8 hours for 14 days Oral antimicrobial therapy consists of Trimethoprim-sulfamethoxazole taken every 12 hours OR Amoxicillin/clavulanic acid (co-amoxiclav) taken every 8 hours for 3 to 6 months
Psittacosis (*Chlamydia psittaci*)		Tetracyclines
Q fever (*Coxiella burnetii*)		Combination of antibiotics including doxycycline, and hydroxychloroquine for several months.
Ricin toxin from *Ricinus communis* (castor beans)		Removal of toxin and supportive care
Staphylococcal enterotoxin B		Bismuth subsalicylate and various antibiotics

Category B Agents	Vaccine	Treatment
Typhus fever (*Rickettsia prowazekii*)		Doxycycline, azithromycin, chloramphenicol, or rifampin.
Viral encephalitis (alphaviruses, such as eastern equine encephalitis, Venezuelan equine encephalitis, and western equine encephalitis)	Some vaccines are available	Supportive care

Category C agents include emerging infectious diseases such as Nipah virus and hantavirus.

These diseases (typical of Ebola and classified as viral hemorrhagic fevers) have periodically caused severe epidemics (see chapter 12 on pandemics for possible examples of this from history). For example, a hantavirus has been put forward as a candidate for several past pandemics, such as the Plague of Athens (430 BC), the Plague of Cyprian (AD 250–271), and the English Sweating Sickness (AD 1485–1551).

Some laboratories must handle these very contagious diseases to study methods of developing both testing systems and vaccines. *The escape of such infectious agents could result in a local if not an international disaster.* Within the United States these laboratories are regulated by the Federal Select Agent Program (FSAP). This program, established in response to a congressional mandate, regulates the possession, use, and transfer of biological select agents and toxins (BSAT) that have the potential to pose a severe threat to public, animal, or plant health, or to animal or plant products. The Federal Select Agent Program is jointly managed by the US Department of Health and Human Services/Centers for Disease Control and Prevention/Center for

Preparedness and Response/Division of Select Agents and Toxins and the US Department of Agriculture/Animal and Plant Health Inspection Service/Veterinary Services/Agriculture Select Agent Services.

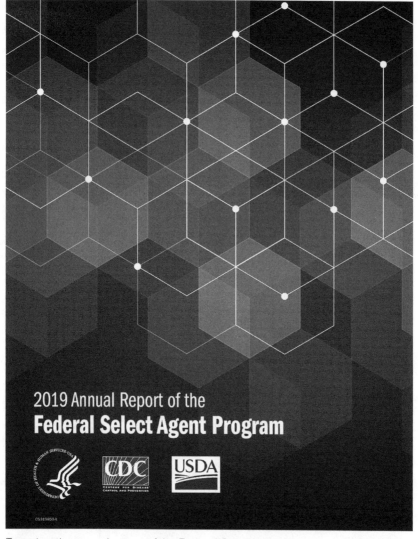

To review the annual report of the Federal State Agent Program, run by the Centers for Disease Control and Prevention and the US Department of Agriculture, visit www.selectagents.gov/index.htm. Any of the links mentioned in this book can be easily accessed by going to the book's website at www.coronacovid19 .com.

Significant Infectious Diseases of the World with a Potential for Epidemics

HHS Select Agents and Toxins

Abrin

Bacillus cereus Biovar
  *anthracis**

Botulinum neurotoxins*

Botulinum neurotoxin producing
  species of *Clostridium**

Conotoxins

Coxiella burnetii

Crimean-Congo hemorrhagic
  fever virus

Diacetoxyscirpenol

Eastern Equine Encephalitis
  virus

Ebola virus*

*Francisella tularensis**

Lassa fever virus

Lujo virus

Marburg virus*

Monkeypox virus

Reconstructed 1918 influenza
  virus

Ricin

Rickettsia prowazekii

SARS-associated coronavirus

Saxitoxin

Chapare

Guanarito

Junin

Machupo

Sabia

Staphylococcal enterotoxins

T-2 toxin

Tetrodotoxin

USDA Select Agents

African horse sickness virus

African swine fever virus

Avian influenza virus

Classical swine fever virus

Coniothyrium glycines (formerly
  Phoma glycinicola and
  Pyrenochaeta glycines)

Foot-and-mouth disease virus*

Goat pox virus

Lumpy skin disease virus

Mycoplasma capricolum

Mycoplasma mycoides

Newcastle disease virus

Peronosclerospora philippinensis
  (Peronosclerospora sacchari)

Peste des petits ruminants virus

Ralstonia solanacearum

Rathayibacter toxicus

Rinderpest virus*

Sclerophthora rayssiae

Sheep pox virus

Swine vesicular disease virus

Synchytrium endobioticum

Xanthomonas oryzae

Overlap Select Agents+

*Bacillus anthracis**

Bacillus anthracis Pasteur strain

Brucella abortus

Brucella melitensis

Brucella suis

*Burkholderia mallei**

HHS Select Agents and Toxins	**USDA Select Agents**
Tick-borne encephalitis complex (flavi) viruses	*Burkholderia pseudomallei*+
Far Eastern subtype	Hendra virus
Siberian subtype	Nipah virus
Kyasanur Forest disease virus	Rift Valley fever virus
Omsk hemorrhagic fever virus	Venezuelan equine encephalitis virus
Variola major virus*	
Variola minor virus*	*Tier 1 agents
*Yersinia pestis**	+These are regulated by both HHS and USDA due to their potential to pose a severe threat to both public health and safety and to animal health or products.
	List last updated on September 24, 2018

According to the report:

In 2019, FSAP received 219 reports of BSAT release and 13 reports of BSAT loss. By comparison, FSAP has received between 193 and 237 reports of releases each year since 2015, and 8 to 12 reports of losses. As in 2015 through 2018, there were again no reports of theft of BSAT in 2019. Of the 219 reports of a BSAT release, 92 were submitted by registered entities and 127 were from nonregistered entities. For registered entities, the most common cause of a release was due to a failure or problem with laboratorian personal protective equipment. For nonregistered laboratories, the most common cause of a release was due to manipulation of BSAT outside of a BSC or other type of equipment designed to protect laboratorians from exposure to infectious aerosols. None of the releases resulted in identified illnesses, deaths, or transmissions among workers or outside of a laboratory.

At least that is the story for the United States during 2019. But the United States, and the world, have not always been so lucky.

- In 1977, a worldwide epidemic of influenza A began in Russia and China, which was eventually traced to a sample of an American strain of flu preserved in a laboratory freezer since 1950.

- In 1978, a hybrid strain of smallpox killed a medical photographer at a lab in Birmingham, England.

- In 2007, live foot-and-mouth diseases leaked from a faulty drainpipe at the Institute for Animal Health in Surry.

- In the United States, "more than 1,100 laboratory incidents involving bacteria, viruses and toxins that pose significant or bioterror risks to people and agriculture were reported to federal regulators during 2008 through 2012," reported *USA Today* in an exposé published in 2014.

- In 2015, the Department of Defense discovered that workers at a germ-warfare testing center in Utah had mistakenly sent close to 200 shipments of live anthrax to laboratories throughout the United States and also to Australia, Germany, Japan, South Korea, and several other countries over the prior twelve years.

Your greatest risk, however, comes not from the weaponized dispersal of a disease, but from nature effectively accomplishing identical results. Included in this group are the diseases listed in Tables 1 and 2 above.

The primary defense against these diseases is to obtain an immunization, if one is available, as indicated in the tables above. Not all of the identified bioterrorism diseases will respond to antibiotics. The most that can be done for many is "supportive care," frequently meaning the use of a respirator and intravenous fluids including specialized cardiac medications. The government stockpiles large quantities of doxycycline and other materials in case of a mass bioterrorism attack. Treatment does not work as well as prevention. We are all familiar with the use of masks, gowns, gloves, and handwashing. And we should be familiar with the importance of immunizations.

IMMUNIZATION PROGRAMS

Examples of successful immunization programs against potentially devastating and currently controlled natural diseases include:

Chickenpox

Chickenpox used to be very common in the United States. In the early 1990s, an average of 4 million people got chickenpox, 10,500 to 13,000 were hospitalized, and 100 to 150 died each year.

The chickenpox vaccine became available in the United States in 1995. Each year, more than 3.5 million cases of chickenpox, 9,000 hospitalizations, and 100 deaths are prevented by chickenpox vaccination in the United States.

Adults who experienced chickenpox as a child are vulnerable to suddenly breaking out with shingles as an adult. The virus is the same, the varicella-zoster virus. Once a person has chickenpox, the virus hides in the nerve ganglion between the spinal cord and the peripheral nerves forever. There is a shingles vaccine for adults to help suppress this painful condition, but ideally everyone has been vaccinated as a child and will not catch chickenpox.

Diphtheria

Before the introduction of vaccines, diphtheria was a leading cause of childhood death around the world, including in the United States. Due to the success of the US immunization program, diphtheria is now nearly unheard of in this country. However, the disease continues to cause illness globally, and there have been outbreaks reported in recent years. In 2018 countries reported more than 16,000 cases of diphtheria to the World Health Organization, and there are likely many more cases.

Hepatitis A

In 2018 there were an estimated 24,900 hepatitis A cases reported in the United States. Since the hepatitis A vaccine was first recommended in 1996, cases of hepatitis A in the United States have declined dramatically. Unfortunately, in recent years the number of people infected has been increasing because there have been multiple outbreaks of hepatitis A in the United States resulting from person-to-person contact, especially among people who use drugs, people experiencing homelessness, and men who have sex with men, and periodically from eating contaminated agricultural products. Vaccination has not kept up with the spread of the disease in the United States.

The hepatitis A vaccine is interesting in that it can provide almost immediate protection from the disease. That is because the virus's incubation period, if it enters your body, is longer than your response to form protective antibodies takes when you receive the vaccine. Almost all injected vaccine requires about 10 days for the body to develop an antibody response. The incubation period for this disease is longer, about 28 days.

Hepatitis B

Worldwide more than 780,000 people per year die from complications of Hepatitis B. In 2018 a total of 3,322 cases of acute (short-term) hepatitis B were reported to the CDC. Since many people may not have symptoms or don't know they are infected, their illness is often not diagnosed. The CDC estimates the actual number of acute hepatitis B cases was closer to 21,600 in 2018. Many more people (about 862,000) are estimated to be living with chronic, long-term hepatitis B. It is estimated 257 million people are living with hepatitis B worldwide. Individuals chronically infected with hepatitis B have a 25 to 40 percent lifetime risk of developing liver cancer.

HIB (*Haemophilus influenza*)

HIB can seriously damage a child's immune system and cause brain damage, hearing loss, or even death. HIB mostly affects children under 5 years old. Before the vaccine, over 20,000 children in the United States were infected each year.

Measles

In the decade before 1963 when a vaccine became available, nearly all children got measles by the time they were 15 years of age. It is estimated 3 to 4 million people in the United States were infected each year. Also, each year among reported cases, an estimated 400 to 500 people died, 48,000 were hospitalized, and 1,000 suffered encephalitis (swelling of the brain) from measles. Since vaccination began in the United States, from year to year, measles cases can range from roughly less than one hundred to a couple hundred. In 2019, 1,282 people from thirty-one states were reported as having measles due to decreases in immunization coverage.

Pertussis (Whooping Cough)
Since 2010, between 15,000 and 50,000 cases of whooping cough were reported each year in the United States, resulting in 20 deaths yearly. Before the whooping cough vaccines were recommended for all infants, about 8,000 people in the United States died each year from whooping cough.

Pneumococcal Disease
This disease is caused by a bacteria called *Streptococcus pneumoniae*. It causes ear infections, sinus infections, pneumonia, and even meningitis, making it very dangerous for children. Vaccines are available for older persons as this disease is a leading cause of death by pneumonia in the older age group. In the United States, it is estimated that more than 150,000 hospitalizations from pneumococcal pneumonia occur each year, and about 5 to 7 percent of those who are hospitalized with it will die. The death rate is even higher in those age 65 and older.

Rotavirus
Rotavirus is contagious and can cause severe watery diarrhea, often with vomiting, fever, and abdominal pain, mostly in infants and young children. Globally, 215,000 child rotavirus deaths accounted for approximately 3.4 percent of all child deaths. Each year, among US children younger than 5 years of age, rotavirus leads to more than 400,000 doctor visits, more than 200,000 emergency room visits, 55,000 to 70,000 hospitalizations, and 20 to 60 deaths. An immunization is available for infants.

Mumps

From January 1 to January 25, 2020, sixteen states in the United States reported mumps infections in seventy people to the CDC. Before the US mumps vaccination program started in 1967, about 186,000 cases were reported each year, but the actual number of cases was likely much higher due to underreporting. A male child catching mumps after puberty has a 40 percent risk of developing this infection in the testes.

Rubella

Before the rubella vaccination program started in 1969, rubella was a common and widespread infection in the United States. During the last major rubella epidemic in the United States from 1964 to 1965, an estimated 12.5 million people got rubella, 11,000 pregnant women lost their babies, 2,100 newborns died, and 20,000 babies were born with congenital rubella syndrome (CRS). Once the vaccine became widely used, the number of people infected with rubella in the United States dropped dramatically.

Today, fewer than ten people in the United States are identified as having rubella each year. Since 2012, all rubella cases had evidence that the individuals were infected when they were living or traveling outside the United States.

SARS-CoV-2

Probably, but this story has not been written yet.

GUESSING THE FUTURE

Oddly enough, an international planning event—what in the military would be considered a wargame—was held in 2019 with international infectious disease specialists, public health officials, and industry leaders to determine what should be involved in a severe pandemic response. It was called "Event 201: A Global Pandemic Exercise" and hosted in New York City on October 18, 2019.

Subsequent to the meeting it was noted that the topic discussed was a theoretical pandemic with a coronavirus. One might have thought it would be about a killer influenza like the 1918 epidemic. Then—almost embarrassingly—out of China comes the very beast they were planning to tame. They wanted to assure the world that the wargame's suggestion that such a virus could probably kill 65 million people was not based on SARS-CoV-2 modeling. So the Center for Health Security came out with the following statement:

Statement about nCoV and our pandemic exercise:

In October 2019, the Johns Hopkins Center for Health Security hosted a pandemic tabletop exercise called Event 201 with partners, the World Economic Forum and the Bill & Melinda Gates Foundation. Recently, the Center for Health Security has received questions about whether that pandemic exercise predicted the current novel coronavirus outbreak in China. To be clear, the Center for Health Security and partners did not make a prediction during our tabletop exercise. For the scenario, we modeled a fictional coronavirus pandemic, but we explicitly stated that it was not a prediction. Instead, the exercise served to highlight preparedness and response challenges that would likely arise in a very severe pandemic. We are not now predicting that the nCoV-2019 outbreak will kill 65 million people. Although our tabletop exercise included a mock novel coronavirus, the inputs we used for modeling the potential impact of that fictional virus are not similar to nCoV-2019.

The recommendations for a worldwide response are remarkably like a worldwide "Operation Warp Speed" or maybe more like a multi-national "War Powers Act" initiative, organizing multi-national heavy lifting for manufacturing personal protective gear, hospital equipment, vaccine development and distribution, testing, and treatment protocol development.

The recommendations of that meeting are attached as Appendix C.

A bioterrorism release of a germ will not collapse civilization, but war and civil collapse frequently cause a massive infectious breakout of the various waterborne diseases, including typhoid fever and cholera. If the government is intact and is trusted during a bioterrorist release, citizens would require and could rely on the expertise of the

CDC and Homeland Security to respond with appropriate guidance and treatment, including a specialized vaccine. In my opinion, we all need to prevent and manage the diseases listed in this book. Prevention is simple, basic, and critical. It consists of proper hygiene (washing hands), water sourcing, food preparation and storage, insect protection, social distancing, mask wearing when appropriate, and immunizations. Beyond the commonly recommended infant, childhood, and adult immunizations, during social breakdown one should consider typhoid, as it commonly explodes during natural disasters.

Civilization can withstand a bioterrorism attack, but it is vulnerable to many natural infections. The best defense is to rapidly access a disease outbreak and to be able to initially isolate it, develop treatments, and finally, formulate prevention strategies, which will almost always rely on immunizations, if they can be developed, and social avoidance (such as sanitation, masks, etc.).

In the end, whether an infectious disease is an endemic disease that is lurking in our backyard and suddenly becomes a pandemic, or whether it is a bioterrorism release or a lab accident, the end result is the same.

Once a disease appears and has spread, it can be dampened only by social engineering (masks, etc.) and can only be reduced significantly or eradicated by the development of herd immunity. That will be gained only by surviving the illness, or immunization.

APPENDIX A

THE GREAT
BARRINGTON DECLARATION

The following is the text of the "Great Barrington Declaration." Please see the discussion presented in chapter 10.

THE GREAT BARRINGTON DECLARATION

As infectious disease epidemiologists and public health scientists we have grave concerns about the damaging physical and mental health impacts of the prevailing COVID-19 policies, and recommend an approach we call Focused Protection.

Coming from both the left and right, and around the world, we have devoted our careers to protecting people. Current lockdown policies are producing devastating effects on short- and long-term public health. The results (to name a few) include lower childhood vaccination rates, worsening cardiovascular disease outcomes, fewer cancer screenings and deteriorating mental health—leading to greater excess mortality in years to come, with the working class and younger members of society carrying the heaviest burden. Keeping students out of school is a grave injustice.

Keeping these measures in place until a vaccine is available will cause irreparable damage, with the underprivileged disproportionately harmed.

Fortunately, our understanding of the virus is growing. We know that vulnerability to death from COVID-19 is more than a thousand-fold higher in the old and infirm than the young. Indeed, for children, COVID-19 is less dangerous than many other harms, including influenza.

As immunity builds in the population, the risk of infection to all—including the vulnerable—falls. We know that all populations will eventually reach herd immunity—i.e., the point at which the rate of new infections is stable—and that this can be assisted by (but is not dependent upon) a vaccine. Our goal should therefore be to minimize mortality and social harm until we reach herd immunity.

The most compassionate approach that balances the risks and benefits of reaching herd immunity is to allow those who are at minimal risk of death to live their lives normally to build up immunity to the virus through natural infection, while better protecting those who are at highest risk. We call this Focused Protection.

Adopting measures to protect the vulnerable should be the central aim of public health responses to COVID-19. By way of example, nursing homes should use staff with acquired immunity and perform frequent testing of other staff and all visitors. Staff rotation should be minimized. Retired people living at home should have groceries and other essentials delivered to their home. When possible, they should meet family members outside rather than inside. A comprehensive and detailed list of measures, including approaches to multi-generational households, can be implemented, and is well within the scope and capability of public health professionals.

Those who are not vulnerable should immediately be allowed to resume life as normal. Simple hygiene measures, such as handwashing and staying home when sick should be practiced by everyone to reduce the herd immunity threshold. Schools and universities should be open for in-person teaching. Extracurricular activities, such as sports, should be resumed. Young low-risk adults should work normally, rather than from home. Restaurants and other businesses should open. Arts, music, sport and other cultural activities should resume. People who are more at risk may participate if they wish, while society as a whole enjoys the protection conferred upon the vulnerable by those who have built up herd immunity.

On October 4, 2020, this declaration was authored and signed in Great Barrington, United States, by:

Dr. Martin Kulldorff, professor of medicine at Harvard University, a biostatistician, and epidemiologist with expertise in detecting and monitoring infectious disease outbreaks and vaccine safety evaluations.

Dr. Sunetra Gupta, professor at Oxford University, an epidemiologist with expertise in immunology, vaccine development, and mathematical modeling of infectious diseases.

Dr. Jay Bhattacharya, professor at Stanford University Medical School, a physician, epidemiologist, health economist, and public health policy expert focusing on infectious diseases and vulnerable populations.

APPENDIX B

THE JOHN SNOW MEMORANDUM

The following is the text of the "John Snow Memorandum." Please see the discussion presented in chapter 10.

THE JOHN SNOW MEMORANDUM

Severe acute respiratory syndrome coronavirus 2 (SARS-CoV-2) has infected more than 35 million people globally, with more than 1 million deaths recorded by the World Health Organization as of October 12, 2020. As a second wave of COVID-19 affects Europe, and with winter approaching, we need clear communication about the risks posed by COVID-19 and effective strategies to combat them. Here, we share our view of the current evidence-based consensus on COVID-19.

SARS-CoV-2 spreads through contact (via larger droplets and aerosols), and longer-range transmission via aerosols, especially in conditions where ventilation is poor. Its high infectivity combined with the susceptibility of unexposed populations to a new virus creates conditions for rapid community spread. The infection fatality rate of COVID-19 is several-fold higher than that of seasonal influenza, and infection can lead to persisting illness, including in young, previously healthy people (i.e., long COVID). It is unclear how long protective immunity lasts and, like other seasonal coronaviruses, SARS-CoV-2 is capable of reinfecting people who have already had the disease, but the frequency of reinfection is unknown. Transmission of the virus can be mitigated through physical distancing, use of face coverings, hand and respiratory hygiene, and by avoiding crowds and poorly ventilated spaces. Rapid testing, contact tracing, and isolation are also critical to controlling transmission. The World Health Organization has been advocating for these measures since early in the pandemic.

In the initial phase of the pandemic, many countries instituted lockdowns (general population restrictions, including orders to stay at home and work from home) to slow the rapid spread of the virus. This was essential to reduce mortality, prevent healthcare services from being overwhelmed, and buy time to set up pandemic response systems to suppress transmission following lockdown. Although lockdowns have been disruptive, substantially affecting mental and physical health, and harming the economy, these effects have often been worse in countries that were not able to use the time during and after lockdown to establish effective pandemic control systems. In the absence of adequate provisions to manage the pandemic and its societal impacts, these countries have faced continuing restrictions.

This has understandably led to widespread demoralization and diminishing trust. The arrival of a second wave and the realization of the challenges ahead has led to renewed interest in a so-called herd immunity approach, which suggests allowing a large uncontrolled outbreak in the low-risk population while protecting the vulnerable. Proponents suggest this would lead to the development of infection-acquired population immunity in the low-risk population, which will eventually protect the vulnerable. This is a dangerous fallacy unsupported by scientific evidence.

Any pandemic management strategy relying upon immunity from natural infections for COVID-19 is flawed. Uncontrolled transmission in younger people risks significant morbidity and mortality across the whole population. In addition to the human cost, this would impact the workforce as a whole and overwhelm the ability of healthcare systems to provide acute and routine care.

Furthermore, there is no evidence for lasting protective immunity to SARS-CoV-2 following natural infection, and the endemic transmission that would be the consequence of waning immunity would present a risk to vulnerable populations for the indefinite future. Such a strategy would not end the COVID-19 pandemic but result in recurrent epidemics, as was the case with numerous infectious diseases before the advent of vaccination. It would also place an unacceptable burden on the economy and healthcare workers, many of whom have died from COVID-19 or experienced trauma as a result of having to practice disaster medicine. Additionally, we still do not understand who might suffer from long COVID. Defining who is vulnerable is complex, but even if we consider those at risk of severe illness, the proportion of vulnerable people constitutes as much as 30 percent of the population in some regions. Prolonged isolation of large swathes of the population is practically impossible and highly unethical. Empirical evidence from many countries shows that it is not feasible to restrict uncontrolled outbreaks to particular sections of society. Such an approach also risks further exacerbating the socioeconomic inequities and structural discriminations already laid bare by the pandemic. Special efforts to protect the most vulnerable are essential but must go hand-in-hand with multi-pronged population-level strategies.

Once again, we face rapidly accelerating increase in COVID-19 cases across much of Europe, the USA, and many other countries across the world. It is critical to act decisively and urgently. Effective measures that suppress and control transmission need to be implemented widely, and they must be supported by financial and social programs that encourage community responses and address the inequities that have been amplified by the pandemic. Continuing restrictions will probably be required in the short term, to reduce transmission and fix ineffective pandemic response systems, in order to prevent future lockdowns. The purpose of these restrictions is to effectively suppress SARS-CoV-2 infections to low levels that allow rapid detection of localized outbreaks and rapid response through efficient and comprehensive find, test, trace, isolate, and support systems so life can return to near-normal without the need for generalized restrictions. Protecting our economies is inextricably tied to controlling COVID-19. We must protect our workforce and avoid long-term uncertainty.

Japan, Vietnam, and New Zealand, to name a few countries, have shown that robust public health responses can control transmission, allowing life to return to near-normal, and there are many such success stories. The evidence is very clear: controlling community spread of COVID-19 is the best way to protect our societies and economies until safe and effective vaccines and therapeutics arrive within the coming months.

We cannot afford distractions that undermine an effective response; it is essential that we act urgently based on the evidence.

The John Snow Memorandum *was originally published in* The Lancet *on October 14, 2020.*

APPENDIX C

EVENT 201 RECOMMENDATIONS

This is the text of the "Event 201" project. Please see the discussion at the end of chapter 13.

RECOMMENDATIONS OF EVENT 201

A Call to Action

The next severe pandemic will not only cause great illness and loss of life but could also trigger major cascading economic and societal consequences that could contribute greatly to global impact and suffering. Efforts to prevent such consequences or respond to them as they unfold will require unprecedented levels of collaboration between governments, international organizations, and the private sector. There have been important efforts to engage the private sector in epidemic and outbreak preparedness at the national or regional level.[1,2] However, there are major unmet global vulnerabilities and international system challenges posed by pandemics that will require new robust forms of public-private cooperation to address.

The Event 201 pandemic exercise, conducted on October 18, 2019, vividly demonstrated a number of these important gaps in pandemic preparedness as well as some of the elements of the solutions between the public and private sectors that will be needed to fill them. The Johns Hopkins Center for Health Security, World Economic Forum, and Bill & Melinda Gates Foundation jointly propose the following:

> Governments, international organizations, and businesses should plan now for how essential corporate capabilities will be utilized during a large-scale pandemic. During a severe pandemic, public sector efforts to control the outbreak are likely to become

overwhelmed. But industry assets, if swiftly and appropriately deployed, could help to save lives and reduce economic losses. For instance, companies with operations focused on logistics, social media, or distribution systems will be needed to enable governments' emergency response, risk communications, and medical countermeasure distribution efforts during a pandemic. This includes working together to ensure that strategic commodities are available and accessible for public health response. Contingency planning for a potential operational partnership between government and business will be complex, with many legal and organizational details to be addressed. Governments should work now to identify the most critical areas of need and reach out to industry players with the goal of finalizing agreements in advance of the next large pandemic. The Global Preparedness Monitoring Board would be well positioned to help monitor and contribute to the efforts that governments, international organizations, and businesses should take for pandemic preparedness and response.

Industry, national governments, and international organizations should work together to enhance internationally held stockpiles of medical countermeasures (MCMs) to enable rapid and equitable distribution during a severe pandemic. The World Health Organization (WHO) currently has an influenza vaccine virtual stockpile, with contracts in place with pharmaceutical companies that have agreed to supply vaccines should WHO request them. As one possible approach, this virtual stockpile model could be expanded to augment WHO's ability to distribute vaccines and therapeutics to countries in the greatest need during a severe pandemic. This should also include any available experimental vaccine stockpiles for any WHO R&D Blueprint pathogens to deploy in a clinical trial during outbreaks in collaboration with CEPI, GAVI, and WHO. Other approaches could involve regional stockpiles or bi- or multinational agreements. During a catastrophic outbreak, countries may be reluctant to part with scarce medical resources. A robust international stockpile could therefore help to ensure that low and middle resource settings receive needed supplies regardless of whether they produce such supplies domestically. Countries with national supplies or domestic manufacturing capabilities should commit to donating some supply/product to this virtual stockpile. Countries should support this effort through the provision of additional funding.

Countries, international organizations, and global transportation companies should work together to maintain travel and trade during severe pandemics. Travel and trade are essential to the global economy as well as to national and even local economies, and they should be maintained even in the face of a pandemic. Improved decision-making, coordination, and communications between the public and private sectors, relating to risk, travel advisories, import/export restrictions, and border measures will be needed. The fear and uncertainty experienced during past outbreaks, even those limited to a national or regional level, have sometimes led to unjustified border measures, the closure of customer-facing businesses, import bans, and the cancellation of airline flights and international shipping. A particularly fast-moving and lethal pandemic could therefore result in political decisions to slow or stop movement of people and goods, potentially harming economies already vulnerable in the face of an outbreak. Ministries of Health and other government agencies should work together now with international airlines and global shipping companies to develop realistic response scenarios and start a contingency planning process with the goal of mitigating economic damage by maintaining key travel and trade routes during a large-scale pandemic. Supporting continued trade and travel in such an extreme circumstance may require the provision of enhanced disease control measures and personal protective equipment for transportation workers, government subsidies to support critical trade routes, and potentially liability protection in certain cases. International organizations including WHO, the International Air Transport Association, and the International Civil Aviation Organization should be partners in these preparedness and response efforts.

Governments should provide more resources and support for the development and surge manufacturing of vaccines, therapeutics, and diagnostics that will be needed during a severe pandemic. In the event of a severe pandemic, countries may need population-level supplies of safe and effective medical countermeasures, including vaccines, therapeutics, and diagnostics. Therefore, the ability to rapidly develop, manufacture, distribute, and dispense large quantities of MCMs will be needed to contain and control a global outbreak. Countries with enough resources should greatly increase this capability. In coordination with WHO, CEPI, GAVI, and other relevant multilateral and domestic mechanisms, investments should be made in new technologies and industrial approaches that will allow concomitant distributed manufacturing. This will require addressing legal and regulatory barriers among other issues.

Global business should recognize the economic burden of pandemics and fight for stronger preparedness. In addition to investing more in preparing their own companies and industries, business leaders and their shareholders should actively engage with governments and advocate for increased resources for pandemic preparedness. Globally, there has been a lack of attention and investment in preparing for high-impact pandemics, and business is largely not involved in existing efforts. To a significant extent this is due to a lack of awareness of the business risks posed by a pandemic. Tools should be built that help large private sector companies visualize business risks posed by infectious disease and pathways to mitigate risk through public-private cooperation to strengthen preparedness. A severe pandemic would greatly interfere with workforce health, business operations, and the movement of goods and services.[3] A catastrophic-level outbreak can also have profound and long-lasting effects on entire industries, the economy, and societies in which business operates. While governments and public health authorities serve as the first line of defense against fast-moving outbreaks, their efforts are chronically under-funded and lack sustained support. Global business leaders should play a far more dynamic role as advocates with a stake in stronger pandemic preparedness.

International organizations should prioritize reducing economic impacts of epidemics and pandemics. Much of the economic harm resulting from a pandemic is likely to be due to counterproductive behavior of individuals, companies, and countries. For example, actions that lead to disruption of travel and trade or that change consumer behavior can greatly damage economies. In addition to other response activities, an increase in and reassessment of pandemic financial support will certainly be needed in a severe pandemic as many sectors of society may need financial support during or after a severe pandemic, including healthcare institutions, essential businesses, and national governments. Furthermore, the ways in which these existing funds can now be used are limited. The International Health Regulations prioritize both minimizing public health risks and avoiding unnecessary interference with international traffic and trade. But there will also be a need to identify critical nodes of the banking system and global and national economies that are too essential to fail—there are some that are likely to need emergency international financial support as well. The World Bank, the International Monetary Fund, regional development banks, national governments, foundations, and others should explore ways to increase the amount and availability of funds in a pandemic and ensure that they can be flexibly used where needed.

Governments and the private sector should assign a greater priority to developing methods to combat mis- and disinformation prior to the next pandemic response. Governments will need to partner with traditional and social media companies to research and develop nimble approaches to countering misinformation. This will require developing the ability to flood media with fast, accurate, and consistent information. Public health authorities should work with private employers and trusted community leaders such as faith leaders, to promulgate factual information to employees and citizens. Trusted, influential private-sector employers should create the capacity to readily and reliably augment public messaging, manage rumors and misinformation, and amplify credible information to support emergency public communications. National public health agencies should work in close collaboration with WHO to create the capability to rapidly develop and release consistent health messages. For their part, media companies should commit to ensuring that authoritative messages are prioritized and that false messages are suppressed including though the use of technology.

Accomplishing the above goals will require collaboration among governments, international organizations, and global business. If these recommendations are robustly pursued, major progress can be made to diminish the potential impact and consequences of pandemics. We call on leaders in global business, international organizations, and national governments to launch an ambitious effort to work together to build a world better prepared for a severe pandemic.

NOTES

1. Global Health Security: Epidemics Readiness Accelerator World Economic Forum. https://www.weforum.org/projects/managing-the-risk-and -impact-of-future-epidemics. Accessed 11/19/19.

2. Private Sector Roundtable. Global Health Security Agenda. https:// ghsagenda.org/home/joining-the-ghsa/psrt/. Accessed 11/19/19.

3. Peter Sands. Outbreak readiness and business impact: protecting lives and livelihoods across the global economy. World Economic Forum 2019. https://www.weforum.org/whitepapers/outbreak-readiness-and-business -impact-protecting-lives-and-livelihoods-across-the-global-economy. Accessed 12/5/19.

This report can be found at www.centerforhealthsecurity.org/ event201/recommendations.html.

APPENDIX D

YEAR 1582 MANUAL
FOR SOCIAL DISTANCING

Reproduced here is a translation of the frequently quoted document from 1582 describing the "best practices" for handling an epidemic devised at that time. While some of it is medieval nonsense, due to not understanding how infectious disease spread, they did come up with a number of valid preventions based upon hundreds of years of experience in surviving epidemics.

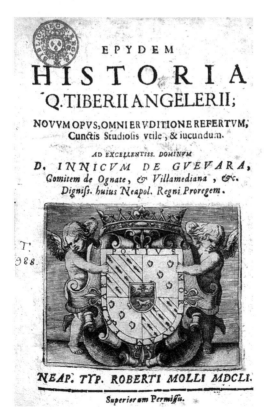

SOCIAL DISTANCING AND QUARANTINE INSTRUCTIONS FROM 1582

Table 1

Sanitary measures described in the original text, *Ectypa Pestilentis Status Algheriae Sardiniae* (1588), by the *Protomedicus* Quinto Tiberio Angelerio (1532–1617)*

No.	Instructions
I	Because the disease is considered a divine punishment, fasts, prayers, vows, and good actions are prescribed to appease the wrath of God.
II	The town must be divided into 10 wards. Each ward must be controlled by a Health Deputy, a person with a high reputation who is invested with full powers. The Health Deputies have the power and the means to 1) punish disobedient citizens without the need to ask for any Magistrate's advice; 2) set fire to all objects suspected to be infected with plague; 3) close the houses in which plague casualties had occurred; and 4) provide the guards and adopt any mandatory measure needed to guarantee the public health.
III	Through edicts, the population must be warned that citizens who do not declare new plague cases—cases that occur in their houses and in other houses—within 6 hours will be prosecuted.
IV	It is strictly forbidden to have contact with a person suspected to have contracted plague before a physician has ruled out the suspicion.
V	The plague hospital must be kept closed by establishing strict guards, thus avoiding the risk that plague patients will mingle with the rest of the population. All patients will be provided all supplies and medicine needed.
VI	The Health Deputies and the *Morbers* must gather twice a day in the so-called "City House" to follow the course of the epidemic and to transmit the information to the Councilors who are assisted by the physicians.

No.	Instructions
VII	Fire must be set to mattresses, fittings, and furniture from all houses in which plague cases have been registered.
VIII	If paupers become ill of a "common" disease and do not want to leave their houses, the city government must provide them with the supplies and medicine that are commonly guaranteed in the hospital.
IX	Meetings, dances, and entertainments are strictly forbidden.
X	When a person is suspected to have died of plague, the corpse must be checked by physicians or surgeons to establish whether the deceased person actually died of plague. If the cause of the death is indeed plague, the relatives of the deceased person must carry the corpse in the courtyard or leave it outside the door.
XI	Two secluded infirmaries must be chosen where persons with plague or suspected to have plague can be isolated. Until these sites are assigned, these persons will be allowed to live in their own houses. However, they should keep themselves separate from the rest of their families as much as possible. Guards will watch over their houses.
XII	Gravediggers should be selected from among persons who had contracted and survived plague during a previous outbreak in another town. Gravediggers must live separately from the rest of the community and far from the hospital. They are not allowed to leave their houses unless accompanied by a Health Deputy.
XIII	Furniture and fittings that are not used must be put aside so that they do not get infected; this will occur until the whole city undergoes disinfection.
XIV	The Councilors and the Jurors of the city of Barcelona (with whom the city has many commercial exchanges) must be immediately informed that a plague outbreak is occurring in Alghero.
XV	Selling entrails of old animals, meat from ill animals, pool fishes, and any other kind of low-quality meat is forbidden.

No.	Instructions
XVI	Each day, the *Morbers* and the physicians are compelled to visit all houses suspected to have plague patients and to arrange the hospitalization of these persons into the isolation center (*tancat*).
XVII	Persons from a house with persons suspected to have plague are forbidden to leave their premises to reach the core of the city. The *Morbers* are charged to fulfill their needs.
XVIII	If plague affects a person living in a house suspected to have persons with plague, gravediggers must take the patient to the hospital or to the isolation place by moving him/her and the bed in which he/she lies. Leaving a plague patient in his/her own house is absolutely forbidden. The transfer to the *tancat* has to take place immediately. If the patient is a distinguished person, he is allowed to stay in his own house.
XIX	A red cross must be painted on the doors of houses known or suspected to have persons with plague so that the rest of the population will keep its distance.
XX	The surgeons are not allowed to leave the hospital or the isolation center. They are allowed to leave those structures only to assist other plague patients, and they must be accompanied by the *Morbers* and the guards.
XXI	Trustworthy persons must be elected to stay in the isolation center and to assist plague patients.
XXII	The pharmacists must provide the poorest with the necessary treatments. A list of the supplied treatments and a list of the citizens must be kept to distinguish between the poorer and the richer. The richer will pay for their treatments, and the city government will pay for the paupers.
XXIII	The city must be cleaned every week from rags and dead things; leather not tanned and rotten raw wool must be put in isolated places; turkeys and cats must be killed and thrown in the sea.
XXIV	It is compulsory to use the Armenian bole for the disinfection of wells and wine casks. Every month, a

No.	Instructions
	sack of Armenian bole must be poured in each well. A certain amount also must be added to the wine casks so that they are preserved from the bad quality and corruption of the plague humors.[1]
XXV	A good supply of wood must be provided to light fires in the city and in the houses during the days and nights. Persons must wear perfumes to eliminate or to mitigate the bad quality of the corrupted air.
XXVI	Fire must be set to the infected objects with no peculiar value. High-value furniture must be washed; exposed to the wind; or even better, disinfected in dry heated stoves/ovens.
XXVII	Frequent inventories must be carried out in the pharmacies to guarantee a large stock of medicines and their availability.
XXVIII	Proclamations must be performed to prevent the citizens from going out of their premises and not move from one house to another. It is forbidden to set fire to furniture and fittings without the respective permission. Those not complying with these instructions will be prosecuted.
XXIX	Bells must be rung and cannon balls and artillery fired to purify the air.
XXX	When the physicians diagnose a new plague case, the *Morbers* must be immediately alerted. They will have the custody of the patient and will take care of him/her.
XXXI	It is compulsory to shut the windows and close the doors of all houses when a person with plague or suspected to have plague is taken to the *tancat* or to the *lazaretto* or when a person who died of plague is taken to the cemetery. Perfumes must be worn and bells must be rung so that the citizens pay attention not to contract the bad air (*disaura*) and, hence, the contagion.
XXXII	It is mandatory to bury plague victims within 6 hours after their death. The corpses must be buried in secluded cemeteries. Long and deep trenches must be excavated, and the corpses must be covered with lime to avoid the air corruption and mephitic vapors. It

No.	Instructions
	is forbidden to bury plague victims inside the churches. Citizens who die outside the city walls must be buried in secluded areas.
XXXIII	During the Mass, it is highly recommended to be careful when shaking hands in token of peace.
XXXIV	The beggars and the homeless must be kept outside the city walls during the day to reduce as much as possible their contact with other citizens.
XXXV	All citizens are compelled not to leave their houses. Only 1 member per household is allowed to go out for shopping. Permission to go out has to be granted by the *Morber* of the area.
XXXVI	People allowed to go out must bear with them a cane measuring 6 feet long. It is mandatory that people keep this distance from one another.
XXXVII	Physicians are compelled to visit all patients. The richest will pay in due time, and the city Councilors will provide for the poorest.
XXXVIII	A large rail, called *parabanda,* must be positioned in front of the counters in the shops in which meat, bread, wine, and foodstuff are sold so that citizens will keep their distance from the counter itself.
XXXIX	It is mandatory to keep dry stoves/ovens always on. These stoves/ovens are similar to those used to cook the flat tiles (*rejolas*). The oven's chamber must be filled with infected textiles/objects after those ones have been washed under the *Morbers'* supervision. The chamber must be constantly heated by an underlying lighted fire.
XL	To allow people to confess, 3-window portable confessionals must be prepared. Two windows are positioned laterally and 1 anteriorly so that the confessor is not reached by the patients' bad breath. For the confessor's sake, the confessional must be perfumed and kept locked in a chapel not accessible to the common people. When sacraments are administered, the confessional must be transported by the gravediggers directly at the patient's bedside and must be taken immediately back to the chapel.

No.	Instructions
XLI	The weekly Head of the *Morbers* is charged to list all the things entering the *lazaretto* and the *tancat* during the week and to attend to all the patients' needs. Similarly, the *Morbers* are charged to fulfill the needs of persons suspected to have plague who must stay isolated in their own houses and watched over by the guards.
XLII	The weekly Head of the *Morbers* must keep the inventory of all the beds, fittings, and furniture that enter into the *tancat* and the *lazaretto*. Things showing a good state of preservation will be used to fulfill the patients' needs, whereas the rest will be burned to avoid the spread of contagion and to avoid robberies.
XLIII	Citizens are forbidden to attempt to cure themselves in their own premises. All ill persons and persons suspected to have plague must be carried to the *tancat* or to the *lazaretto*. Guards must accompany these persons and keep other citizens away during the transfer.
XLIV	All infected textiles and objects from the *lazaretto* must undergo laundry and then disinfection in the dry oven.
XLV	During summertime, bonfires must be set in wooden areas to purify the air taking care not to damage the land's owners.
XLVI	Infected infants who are orphans or do not have a wet nurse must be bottle fed by using the milk of well-fed goats. For this purpose, goats will be allowed to live inside the *lazaretto*.
XLVII	The buboes of plague patients must be cut open or cauterized. Those who are reluctant must be tied so that surgeons can intervene.
XLVIII	People suspected to be infected and convalescents must undergo quarantine before they are allowed to get back in contact with healthy inhabitants.
XLIX	When the plague epidemic is close to its end, a high number of male and female goats will have to be introduced within the city walls during the night. The animals will be placed inside the houses of the plague patients, and this operation will be repeated for several

No.	Instructions
	nights. However, for the population's sake, the houses also will undergo whitewashing. Whitewashing will be performed by painters who survived the contagion. For the less suspected houses, it is required that the windows be kept wide open and that perfumes be sprayed and all surfaces washed with vinegar.
L	People living in the surroundings are forbidden to enter the city walls unless their health status has been carefully checked and permission from the *Morbers* granted. The *Morbers* are entrusted to check that these persons' belongings be washed and disinfected in the oven. Once these persons have been proved to be healthy, they will be admitted to live in their new houses but only after their own disinfection. Once they have settled down in their new houses, these persons are compelled to stay isolated from the rest of the population for some days.
LI	The houses' owners and the lodgers are compelled to disinfect, whitewash, ventilate, and water their residences. In case they do not attend the task, the city government will have to bear the costs.
LII	It is strictly forbidden to sell linen, silk, cotton, and wool textiles without permission from the *Morber* of the area.
LIII	The *Morbers* are compelled to carry out the complete disinfection of the city afterward and house after house. The darkest houses and those lacking aeration will be whitewashed, perfumed, and cleaned with vinegar. Bonfires will be set all around. Similar precautions will be applied to the houses whose walls are covered with golden slivers and leathers. Silk, cotton, linen, and woolly textiles must be washed and disinfected in the oven.
LIV	Once all these precautions have been taken, the Councilors, the Deputies, the hospital attendants, and the physician Angelerio himself [the other anonymous physician had already died of the plague] must visit all

No.	Instructions
	the Alghero inhabitants, house after house. The citizens will be asked under oath if the *Morbers* had indeed disinfected their houses properly. In case disinfection had not properly been performed, another will be carried out within the following 6 days.
LV	It is compulsory that all citizens expose to the wind the furniture and fittings from their houses for 10 days. When the Counselors visit the citizens, at the end of the epidemic, everything must be in order.
LVI	Each citizen who is aware that his neighbors have not carried out the disinfection properly must notify it to the Councilors and *Morbers*. The latter will keep the secret and will pay the honest citizen with a money consideration.
LVII	It is compulsory to disinfect the *tancat* and the *lazaretto* located outside the city walls by using the same methods described in Instruction LIII. Fire must be set to every object kept inside the above structures. The persons who have survived and complied with the quarantine will be allowed to return to the city wearing new and disinfected clothes. The main city hospital, Sant' Antonio, must be disinfected and reordered. The hospital will be reopened to all the population and will go back to its standard use.

Morbers: the health or plague guardians. The *Morbers*' task was to watch over the sanitary conditions of the ships docking at the island's harbors and assist the *Protomedicus* during the plague outbreaks. The usual *Morbers*' duties were largely extended during the 1582–1583 plague outbreak.

Tancat: isolation center for persons suspected of having plague.

Lazaretto: isolation center for plague patients.

APPENDIX E

GLOSSARY OF
EPIDEMIOLOGICAL TERMS

Acute condition: the abrupt onset of illness or disease with a brief duration (three months) that is rapidly progressive and in need of urgent care or serious enough to alter behavior.

Agent: a factor whose presence, or in the case of deficiency diseases, relative absence is essential for the occurrence of a disease.

Age-specific rate: a rate categorized by age group that is determined by dividing the number of individuals in the age group within the population by the number of occurrences in that age group.

Airborne transmission: transmission that occurs when infectious agents are carried by dust suspended in the air. With airborne transmission, direct contact is not needed to spread disease (as compared with respiratory droplet transmission). Infection may be transmitted over short distances by large droplets, and at longer distances by droplet nuclei generated by coughing and sneezing.

Analytic epidemiology: a search for cause and effect by quantifying the association between exposures and outcomes and testing hypotheses about causal relationships.

Analytic study: a comparative study concerned with identifying or measuring the effects of risk factors or with the health effects of specific exposures.

Association: a state in which two attributes occur together either more or less often than expected by chance.

Attack rate: the risk of contracting an illness during a specified period, with the overall attack rate equaling the total number of new cases divided by the total at-risk population.

Average length of stay: the sum of inpatient days divided by the number of patient admissions with the same diagnosis-related group classification.

Bias: a deviation of results or inferences from the truth.

Biologic transmission: occurs when the vector consumes the agent, often through a blood meal from an infected animal, replicates and/or develops it, and then regurgitates the pathogen onto or injects it into a susceptible animal.

Carrier: a person or animal that shows no symptoms of a disease but harbors the genetic mutation associated with that disease and is capable of transmitting it to others.

Case: A countable instance of a particular disease or condition within the population or study group.

Case-control study: an observational analytic study based on the presence or absence of disease.

Case definition: a set of standard criteria for classifying whether a person has a particular disease, syndrome, or other health condition, which must include the three classical dimensions of epidemiological variables: time, place, and person.

Case-fatality rate: the proportion of individuals with a particular condition who die from that condition; calculated by dividing the number of incident cases by the number of cause-specific deaths among those cases.

Case report study: the detailed profile of an individual patient.

Case series study: a type of medical research study describing the characteristics of a number of patients with a given disease (also known as a clinical series).

Cause of disease: a factor that directly influences the occurrence of disease.

Chain of infection: a process beginning when an infectious agent leaves its reservoir or host through a portal of exit, is passed along through direct, indirect, or airborne transmission, and enters into a susceptible host.

Clade: a group of biological taxa (such as a species) that includes all descendants of one common ancestor.

Clinical trial: experimental research studies aimed at evaluating medical, surgical, or behavioral intervention for the sake of determining a potential cure.

Cluster: a group of cases of a disease or health-related conditions closely connected in time and place.

Cohort: a well-defined group of people sharing a common experience or exposure who are then followed up for incidence of new diseases or events.

Cohort study: an observational analytic study. Inclusion is based on exposure characteristics or membership in a group, and health outcomes are then identified and evaluated.

Colonized: a carrier state occurring when a noninfected person has the infectious agent on their skin.

Common source outbreak: an outbreak resulting from a group of persons being exposed to an infectious agent or toxin.

Communicable disease: a disease capable of direct or indirect transmission from one person to another.

Contact: exposure to a contagious disease often through close association with an infected individual.

Contagious: capable of spreading disease from one person to another through direct or indirect transmission.

Control: a comparison group of individuals in a case-control study who do not have the disease or condition being studied.

Crude mortality rate: a mortality rate from all causes of death for a population.

Cross-sectional study: the study of a set of individuals who are studied either at a single point in time or over a defined period of time for the prevalence of disease.

Death-to-case ratio: the number of deaths associated with a particular disease during a specified time period divided by the number of new cases of that disease identified during the same period.

Descriptive epidemiology: the organizing and summarizing of health-related data according to time, place, and person.

Determinant: any factor that brings about change in a health condition or other specified characteristics.

Direct transmission: the immediate transfer of an infectious agent from a reservoir to a susceptible host by direct contact or through droplet spread. Such diseases are unlikely to survive for significant periods of time away from a host, as they require physical contact between an infected and susceptible person.

Distribution: the frequency and pattern of health-related characteristics and events in a population.

Droplet: a particle of moisture discharged when coughing, sneezing, or speaking.

Droplet spread: the direct transmission of an infectious agent by spraying relatively large, short-ranged droplets or aerosols produced when sneezing, coughing, or talking.

Ecological study: a study involving the comparison of disease frequency between different populations based on one or more risk factors of interest (also known as a correlational study).

Endemic disease: the constant presence or usual prevalence of a disease within a certain population group or geographic region.

Environmental factor: third part of the epidemiologic triad bringing the other two parts (the host and agent) together in order for disease to occur.

Epidemic: the occurrence of more cases of disease than expected in a given area or among a specific group of people over a particular period of time.

Epidemic curve: a histogram showing the course of an outbreak or epidemic by plotting the number of cases by time of onset.

Epidemic period: a period of time when the number of reported disease cases is greater than expected.

Epidemiologic triad: the traditional model of infectious disease causation, which includes three components: an external agent, a susceptible host, and an environment that brings the host and agent together so that disease occurs.

Epidemiology: a study of the factors that impact the health and illness of a population.

Evaluation: a process that attempts to determine as systematically and objectively as possible the relevance, effectiveness, and impact of activities in the light of their objectives.

Exposed (group): a group whose members have been exposed to a supposed cause of disease or health condition of interest, or who possess a characteristic that is a determinant of the health outcome of interest.

Fecal-oral transmission: the passing of pathogens in fecal particles to the mouth of another person; most commonly the result of ingesting contaminated food or water or improper hygiene practices.

Fomite: an object such as a telephone, doorknob, or article of clothing that may be contaminated with infectious agents (such as bacteria, parasites, or viruses) and serve in their transmission.

Frequency distribution: the arrangement of statistical data in order of the frequency of each size of the variable.

Health: a complete state of physical, mental, and social well-being and not solely the absence of disease.

Health information system: a collection of statistics from multiple sources used to derive information pertaining to various aspects of health (health care, health status, health provision and use of services, and impact on health).

High-risk group: a group within a community with an elevated risk of disease.

Host: any living organism with the ability to be infected by an infectious agent under normal conditions.

Host factor: an inherent factor (age, race, sex, behaviors, etc.) influencing an individual's susceptibility, exposure, or response to a causative agent.

Hyperendemic disease: disease exhibiting a high and continued incidence rate.

Hypothesis: a supposition arrived at from observation or reflection; any assumption provided in such a way that will allow it to be tested and refuted.

Immune: denotes those who show no clinical signs of infection following exposure to a pathogen.

Immunity, active: the resistance developed in response to stimulus by an antigen (infecting agent or vaccine); often characterized by the presence of antibody produced by the host.

Immunity, herd: a group's resistance to the spread of an infectious agent as a result of the higher number of individuals within the group being immune to the agent.

Immunity, passive: immunity conferred by an antibody produced in another host acquired either naturally from mother to infant or artificially through administration of an antibody-containing preparation (antiserum or immune globulin).

Incidence rate: measure of frequency with which an illness or similar event occurs in a population over a period of time; calculated by dividing the at-risk population with the number of new cases occurring during a given time period.

Incubation period: time from disease exposure to onset of symptoms of infectious disease.

Index case: the initial case to come to the attention of a disease investigator. Identification of the index case can be helpful in determining the origin of the disease's outbreak.

Indirect transmission: the passing of a disease from a previously uninfected person or group after coming in contact with a contaminated surface.

Infectivity: the proportion of individuals exposed to an infectious agent who become infected by it.

Inference, statistical: the development of generalizations from sample data, often with calculated degrees of uncertainty.

International classification of disease (ICD): the diagnostic classification standard for all clinical and research purposes; established for the sake of promoting international comparability in the collection, classification, processing, and presentation of health statistics.

Latency period: time between exposure and showing symptoms of disease.

Life expectancy: the average number of years a person is expected to live.

Measure of association: a quantified relationship between exposure and disease.

Measure of central location: a single value representing the entire distribution of data.

Measure of dispersion: a measure of the spread of a distribution out from its central value.

Median: the middle value in a distribution above and below which lie an equal number of values.

Medical surveillance: an effort to detect early symptoms of a disease by monitoring potentially exposed individuals.

Midrange: the midpoint within a set of observations.

Misclassification: an error in classifying subjects by disease or risk factor distorting associations between disease and risk factors.

Mode: the most frequently occurring value in a distribution.

Mortality rate: the ratio between deaths and individuals in a specified population and during a particular time period.

Mortality rate, infant: the number of infant deaths (those who die before their first birthday) for every 1,000 births.

Mortality rate, neonatal: the number of children less than 28 days of age who die divided by the number of live births that year.

Mortality rate, postneonatal: the number of newborns in a specified geographic area dying between 28 and 364 days of age.

Natural history of disease: the progression of a disease process in an individual over time.

Necessary cause: the presence of a causal factor for the occurrence of the effect of disease.

Normal curve: a bell-shaped curve resulting from normal distribution.

Normal distribution: a symmetrical distribution of scores with the majority concentrated around the mean.

Observational study: a study in situations where nature is allowed to take its course. These are often a cause of inaccurate inferences and are low-grade studies. Many initial treatments shown as possible from observational studies do not prove of value or are even harmful when placebo-controlled, double-blind studies are performed.

Odds ratio: the chance of an event occurring in one group compared to that of another group.

Outbreak: a localized as opposed to generalized epidemic (synonymous with epidemic).

Pandemic: an epidemic affecting a large portion of the population over a wide area (several countries or continents).

Pathogenicity: infected individuals who then develop clinical disease after exposure to a causative agent.

Period prevalence: prevalence measured over an interval of time; the proportion of persons with a particular disease or attribute at any time during the interval.

Person-time rate: the number of new cases of disease during a specified time interval.

Point prevalence: the proportion of the population with a given disease or condition at a specific point in time.

Prevalence: the proportion of cases, events, or conditions in a given population.

Prevalence rate: the proportion of the population with a given disease or condition at a specific point in time or over a specific time period.

Propagated outbreak: an outbreak lacking a common source, spreading instead from person to person.

Proportion: an equation that defines that two given ratios are equivalent to each other. The proportion states the equality of the two fractions or ratios.

Proportionate mortality: the proportion of deaths in a specified population over a period of time attributable to different causes.

Prospective study: a study in which the participants are identified and then followed forward in time.

Race-specific mortality rate: a mortality rate defined by a specified racial group.

Random sample: a population sample derived by selecting individuals such that each has the same probability of selection; meant to be an unbiased representation of a group.

Rate: the frequency with which an event occurs in a defined population.

Rate ratio: a relative difference measure used to compare the incidence rates of events occurring at any given point in time.

Recall bias: a systematic error caused by the inaccuracy or incompleteness of the recollections retrieved by study participants regarding events or experiences from the past.

Relative risk: a measure of the risk of a certain event happening in one group compared to the risk of the same event happening in another group.

Reliability: consistency of a measurement repeated on the same subjects.

Representative sample: characteristics of a sample corresponding to those of the original or reference population.

Reservoir: a person, animal, plant, soil, or substance in which an infectious agent normally lives and multiplies.

Retrospective study: a study looking backward in time after both the exposure and outcome of interest has occurred.

Risk: the probability of a disease or event occurring.

Risk factor: something that increases a person's chances for developing a disease. This could be personal behavior, environmental exposure, or an inherited characteristic associated with an increased occurrence of disease.

Risk ratio: a measure of the risk of a certain event happening in one group compared to the risk of the same event happening in another group.

Sample: a selected population subset that may be random or nonrandom and representative or nonrepresentative.

Seasonality: seasonal patterns impacting change in physiological status or disease occurrence.

Secular trend: changes over an extended period of time, usually years or decades.

Sensitivity: the ability of a test or system to detect fluctuation in disease occurrence.

Sex-specific mortality rate: a mortality rate identified as different due to male or female gender.

Skewed: asymmetrical distribution.

Source: the person, animal, or object from which an infection is acquired.

Specificity: the proportion of disease-free individuals correctly identified as not having disease by a screening test or case definition.

Sporadic: an infrequent or irregular occurrence of a disease.

Spot map: a map indicating the location of each case of a rare disease potentially relevant to the health event being investigated.

Standard deviation: a measure of dispersion of a frequency distribution, equal to the positive square root of the variance.

Standard error (of the mean): defines how accurate the mean of any given sample from that population is likely to be compared to the true population mean.

Sufficient cause: an etiological factor guaranteeing that the result in question will occur.

Survival curve: graph of survival probability versus time; often used to present the results of clinical trials.

Table: data arranged in rows and columns.

Table shell: the framework of a table prior to any data entry.

Transmission of infection: means by which an infectious agent spreads through the environment or to other individuals. The two types of transmission are direct transmissions, spread through human contact, and indirect transmissions, spread from one person to another through an intermediary agent (e.g., air or water, a contaminated surface, or a living disease vector).

Trend: the inclination to proceed in a certain direction at a certain rate over a long period of time for the sake of defining the course of a symptom, disease, or method of disease management.

Universal precautions: a CDC-issued approach to infection control to treat all human blood and certain human body fluids as if they were known to be infectious for HIV, HBV, and other blood-borne pathogens.

Usual source of care: a provider or place a patient most frequently visits when ill or seeking medical advice, such as a general practice.

Validity: the extent to which the findings of an investigation reflect the truth.

Variance: a measure of dispersion within a set of observations defined by the sum of squares of deviations from the mean, divided by the number of degrees of freedom in the set of observations; in other words, a lot of difference in results may allow a trend to be identified, but if there is a lot of variance this trend would be questionable.

Vector: animals capable of transmitting diseases. Mosquitoes, flies, ticks, fleas, mites, rats, and dogs are all examples of vectors. The mobility of vectors as well as changes in vector behavior impact the transmission range and pattern of a disease. This makes it crucial to study both the vector and the disease-causing microorganism in order to establish a proper method of disease prevention.

Vector-borne transmission: the indirect transmission of an agent carried from a reservoir to a susceptible host. While mosquitoes are most commonly associated with vector-borne transmissions, diseases can also be spread through the feces of a vector or microorganisms located on the outside surface of a vector (such as a fly) coming in contact with food, a common touch surface, or a susceptible individual.

Vehicle: an inanimate substance by or on which an infected agent passes to a susceptible host. Some examples include food, clothing, dust, or instruments.

Virulence: the proportion of individuals with a clinical disease who become severely ill or die following infection.

Vital statistics: data relating to births, marriages, divorces, and deaths based on registration of such vital events.

Years of potential life lost: a measure of the impact on a population caused by premature mortality; the sum of the differences between a predetermined/desired life span and the age of death for those who died before that predetermined age.

Zoonoses: the transmission of an infectious disease from animals to humans under normal conditions.

NOTES

CHAPTER 1

1. Tuitem A. S., and Fisman, D. N., "Reporting, Epidemic Growth, and Reproduction Numbers for the 2019 Novel Coronavirus (2019-nCoV) Epidemic," *Annals of Int Med* (Feb. 2020), https://doi.org/10.7326/M20-0358.

2. Phipps, S. J., Grafton, R. Q., and Kompas, T., "Robust estimates of the true (population) infection rate for COVD-19: A backcasting approach," *R. Soc. Open Sci.* 7:20090, http://dx.doi.org/10.1098/sos.200909.

CHAPTER 2

1. Yesli, R., and Otter, J. (2011), "Minimum Infective Dose of the Major Human Respiratory and Enteric Viruses Transmitted Through Food and the Environment," *Food Environ Virol* 3: 1–30.

2. Gastañaduy, A. S., and Bégué, R. E. (2017), "Acute Gastroenteritis Viruses," *Infectious Diseases* (4th ed.).

CHAPTER 3

1. "As Christmas Nears, Virus Experts Look for Lessons from Thanksgiving," *New York Times*, www.nytimes.com, December 20, 2020.

CHAPTER 7

1. O'Driscoll, M., et al. (2020), "Age-specific mortality and immunity patterns of SARS-CoV-2," *Nature* 10:1038.

2. *JAMA Network Open* 4(1) (2021):e2033706, doi:10.1001/jamanetworkopen.2020.33706.

3. *New York Times* reported on January 17, 2017, an estimated 23,900,000 cases had resulted in 397,566 deaths.

4. https://ourworldindata.org/identify-covid-exemplars.

5. Yehia, B. R., Winegar, A., Fogel, R., et al., "Association of race with mortality among patients hospitalized with coronavirus disease 2019 (COVID-19) at 92 US hospitals," *JAMA Network Open* 3(8) (2020):e2018039, doi:10.1001/jamanetworkopen.2020.18039.

6. https://covidtracking.com.

7. https://link.springer.com/content/pdf/10.1186/s12916-020-01640-8.pdf.

CHAPTER 8

1. Syomin, B.V., and Ilyin, Y. V. (2019) "Virus-like Particles as an Instrument of Vaccine Production," *Mol. Biol.* 53(3): 323–34.

2. https://www.cdc.gov/vaccinesafety/concerns/adjuvants.html.

3. https://www.cdc.gov/vaccines/pubs/pinkbook/downloads/appendices/B/excipient-table-2.pdf.

4. https://www.who.int/blueprint/priority-diseases/key-action/list-of-candidate-vaccines-developed-against-sars.pdf.

CHAPTER 11

1. *Pys. Fluids* 32.109013 (2020), https:/doi.org/10.1063/5.0025476.

2. Michael Osterholm podcast. https://www.osterholmupdate/podcast/episode/1ao6a8bc/episode-32-stop-swapping-air.

3. htttp://www.siverlon.com.

4. https://www.canada.ca/en/public-health/services/diseases/2019-novel-coronavirus-infection/prevention-risks/sew-no-sew-instructions-non-medical-masks-face-coverings.html last accessed November 22, 2020.

5. https://www.cdc.gov/coronavirus/2019-ncov/prevent-getting-sick/how-to-make-cloth-face-covering.html, last accessed November 23, 2020.

CHAPTER 12

1. https://www.mphonline.org (articles).

2. Universal precautions refer to the technique of treating everyone as if they were contagious, using protective gloves, masks, gowns, washing hands—all techniques we have become familiar in performing due to SARS-CoV-2.

3. Anelerii, Q.T., Ectypus pestilentsis status Algheriae Sardiniae, 1588. Reference doi: http://dx.doi.org/10.3201/eid1909.120311.

APPENDIX D

1. Armenian bole is a natural mixture of hydrated silicate clays colored with red iron oxide.

INDEX

Italicized page numbers note illustrations. Charts, maps, and tables are represented by *c*, *m*, and *t*, respectively.

ABOUT THE AUTHOR

A member of the Board of Trustees of the International Association for Medical Assistance to Travelers (IAMAT), **Dr. Forgey** is a fellow of the Explorer's Club and a fellow of the Academy of Wilderness Medicine. He holds the Certificate in Travel Health (CTH) from the International Society of Travel Medicine. A former captain in the US Army, Infantry, he saw over thirty months' active duty in Vietnam prior to leaving the service and attending medical school at Indiana University. He was awarded the Bronze Star and Army Commendation Medal for his service in Vietnam.

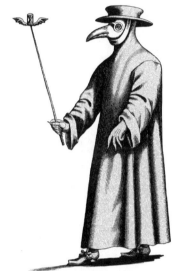

Dr. Forgey has practiced travel medicine for over forty years while attending patients in three hospital systems in northern Indiana. He has made over forty medical service missions to people in rural Haiti and has lectured internationally to physicians as an expert on various medical conditions. He is an International Fellow of the Royal Society of Medicine and a

The medieval plague doctor—dressed not unlike how I feel in clinic often these days.

WIKIMEDIA COMMONS

member of multiple medical associations and societies in the United States, as well as a past president of the Wilderness Medical Society.

All links mentioned in this book are conveniently located at this book's website: www.coronacov19.com.